# Rhinology Handbook

# *Rhinology Handbook*

**Editor**

**Ashutosh Kacker** MD
Professor of Clinical Otolaryngology
Department of Otolaryngology—Head and Neck Surgery
Weill Cornell Medical College
New York, New York, USA

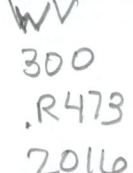

*The Health Sciences Publisher*

Philadelphia | New Delhi | London | Panama

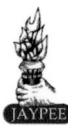 **Jaypee Brothers Medical Publishers (P) Ltd**

**Headquarters**
Jaypee Brothers Medical Publishers (P) Ltd.
4838/24, Ansari Road, Daryaganj
New Delhi 110 002, India
Phone: +91-11-43574357
Fax: +91-11-43574314
E-mail: jaypee@jaypeebrothers.com

**Overseas Offices**

J.P. Medical Ltd.
83, Victoria Street, London
SW1H 0HW (UK)
Phone: +44-20 3170 8910
Fax: +44(0)20 3008 6180
E-mail: info@jpmedpub.com

Jaypee Medical Inc.
325 Chestnut Street
Suite 412
Philadelphia, PA 19106, USA
Phone: +1 267-519-9789
E-mail: support@jpmedus.com

Jaypee Brothers Medical Publishers (P) Ltd.
Bhotahity, Kathmandu, Nepal
Phone: +977-9741283608
E-mail: kathmandu@jaypeebrothers.com

Jaypee-Highlights Medical Publishers Inc.
City of Knowledge, Bld. 237, Clayton
Panama City, Panama
Phone: +1 507-301-0496
Fax: +1 507-301-0499
E-mail: cservice@jphmedical.com

Jaypee Brothers Medical Publishers (P) Ltd.
17/1-B, Babar Road, Block-B, Shaymali
Mohammadpur, Dhaka-1207
Bangladesh
Mobile: +08801912003485
E-mail: jaypeedhaka@gmail.com

Website: www.jaypeebrothers.com
Website: www.jaypeedigital.com

© 2016, Jaypee Brothers Medical Publishers

The views and opinions expressed in this book are solely those of the original contributor(s)/author(s) and do not necessarily represent those of editor(s) of the book.

All rights reserved. No part of this publication may be reproduced, stored or transmitted in any form or by any means, electronic, mechanical, photocopying, recording or otherwise, without the prior permission in writing of the publishers.

All brand names and product names used in this book are trade names, service marks, trademarks or registered trademarks of their respective owners. The publisher is not associated with any product or vendor mentioned in this book.

Medical knowledge and practice change constantly. This book is designed to provide accurate, authoritative information about the subject matter in question. However, readers are advised to check the most current information available on procedures included and check information from the manufacturer of each product to be administered, to verify the recommended dose, formula, method and duration of administration, adverse effects and contraindications. It is the responsibility of the practitioner to take all appropriate safety precautions. Neither the publisher nor the author(s)/editor(s) assume any liability for any injury and/or damage to persons or property arising from or related to use of material in this book.

This book is sold on the understanding that the publisher is not engaged in providing professional medical services. If such advice or services are required, the services of a competent medical professional should be sought.

Every effort has been made where necessary to contact holders of copyright to obtain permission to reproduce copyright material. If any have been inadvertently overlooked, the publisher will be pleased to make the necessary arrangements at the first opportunity.

**Inquiries for bulk sales may be solicited at:** jaypee@jaypeebrothers.com

*Rhinology Handbook*

*First Edition*: **2016**

ISBN: 978-93-5152-775-6

*Printed at: Samrat Offset Pvt. Ltd.*

## Dedicated to

*My father, Dr Santosh Kumar Kacker, who is my role model in my personal and professional life, as well as to my wife, mother, and children, who made this book possible.*

# Contributors

**Seth M Brown** MD MBA FACS
Clinical Assistant Professor
Department of Surgery
Division of Otolaryngology
University of Connecticut School of Medicine
Farmingham, Connecticut, USA

**Angela Donaldson** MD
Atlanta Institute for ENT
Atlanta, Georgia, USA

**James Foshee**
Student
Jefferson Medical College
Thomas Jefferson University
Philadelphia, Pennsylvania, USA

**Qasim Husain** MD
Resident Physician
Department of Otolaryngology—Head and Neck Surgery
New York Presbyterian Hospital—Columbia/Cornell
New York, New York, USA

**Alfred Marc Iloreta** MD
Assistant Professor
Department of Otolaryngology
Mount Sinai School of Medicine
New York, New York, USA

**Ashutosh Kacker** MD
Professor of Clinical Otolaryngology
Department of Otolaryngology—Head and Neck Surgery
Weill Cornell Medical College
New York, New York, USA

**Gurston G Nyquist** MD
Assistant Professor
Department of Otolaryngology
Thomas Jefferson University
Philadelphia, Pennsylvania, USA

**Valeria Silva Merea** MD
Resident Physician
Department of Otolaryngology—Head and Neck Surgery
New York Presbyterian Hospital—Columbia/Cornell
New York, New York, USA

**Karin PQ Oomen** MD PhD
Fellow
Department of Otolaryngology—Head and Neck Surgery
Pediatric Otolaryngology—Head and Neck Surgery
Weill Cornell Medical College
New York, New York, USA

**Roheen Raithatha** MD
Clinical Instructor
Department of Otolaryngology—Head and Neck Surgery
Icahn School of Medicine of Mount Sinai
New York, New York, USA

**Marc R Rosen** MD
Professor of Otolaryngology—Head and Neck Surgery and Neurological Surgery
Sidney Kimmel Medical College at Thomas Jefferson University
Philadelphia, Pennsylvania, USA

**Patrick Stevens** MS MD
Physician
Department of Otolaryngology
University of Connecticut Health Center
Farmington, Connecticut, USA

**Abtin Tabaee** MD
Associate Professor of Otolaryngology
Department of Otolaryngology
Icahn School of Medicine at Mount Sinai
New York, New York, USA

**Belachew Tessema** MD FACS
Assistant Clinical Professor
Connecticut Sinus Institute
University of Connecticut School of Medicine
Farmington, Connecticut, USA

# *Preface*

Disorders of the ear, nose, and throat are highly prevalent in the primary care setting and can have a substantial impact upon the quality of human life. It is therefore imperative to promote education in otolaryngology among primary care providers, especially as diagnostic and treatment modalities undergo continual innovation. The area of rhinology is of particular importance. Diseases of the nose, paranasal sinuses, and skull base are common among the American populace, including allergic rhinitis, acute/chronic sinusitis, nasal obstruction and epistaxis. Successful medical management at the primary care level can usually be achieved with an accurate diagnosis based upon assessment of patient history and nasal symptoms and delivery of an appropriate treatment, such as antibiotics, antihistamines, or decongestants. With an intensifying shortage of otolaryngologists, an aging and expanding population, and increasing health coverage under the Affordable Care Act, primary care providers will continue to take greater roles in managing these illnesses. The goal of this manual is to familiarize primary care physicians, medical students, residents, physician assistants, nurse practitioners, and other healthcare professionals with common rhinological conditions. This comprehensive knowledge will allow primary care providers to effectively diagnose and treat disorders and refer patients to the appropriate otolaryngologist for complicated problems that require more sophisticated diagnostic tools and potential surgical interventions. The authors are confident that continuing education in rhinology will improve the efficiency and quality of American healthcare.

**Ashutosh Kacker**

# *Acknowledgments*

I wish to acknowledge Dr Vijay Anand, who is a guiding force and a mentor to all of us.

I would also like to thank Shri Jitendar P Vij (Group Chairman), Ms Chetna Malhotra Vohra (Associate Director) and Ms Angima Shree (Development Editor) of M/s Jaypee Brothers Medical Publishers (P) Ltd., New Delhi, India, and the Publishing staff of JP Medical, Inc, Philadelphia, PA, USA.

# Contents

1. **Anatomy and Physiology of the Nose, Paranasal Sinuses, and Olfaction** .................... 1
   *Angela Donaldson, Roheen Raithatha*
   - Anatomy of the Olfactory System  *1*
   - Sinonasal Physiology  *6*
   - Embryology of the Nose and Paranasal Sinuses  *8*
   - Anatomy of the Nose and Paranasal Sinuses  *9*

2. **Acute Rhinosinusitis** .................... 25
   *Abtin Tabaee*
   - Pathophysiology  *25*
   - Clinical Presentation and Diagnosis  *27*
   - Therapy  *31*
   - Complications  *33*

3. **Chronic Rhinosinusitis** .................... 39
   *Patrick Stevens, Belachew Tessema, Seth M Brown*
   - Epidemiology  *39*
   - Pathogenesis  *40*
   - Clinical Presentation, Evaluation and Diagnosis  *43*
   - Subtypes of Rhinosinusitis  *46*
   - Management  *48*
   - Complications of Rhinosinusitis  *51*

4. **Nasal Obstruction** .................... 57
   *Qasim Husain, Ashutosh Kacker*
   - Objective Nasal Obstruction  *57*
   - Subjective Nasal Obstruction  *81*
   - Approach to the Patient with Nasal Obstruction  *84*

5. **Nasal Neoplasms** .................... 97
   *Valeria Silva Merea, Ashutosh Kacker*
   - Benign Nasal Neoplasms  *98*
   - Malignant Nasal Neoplasms  *101*

6. **Epistaxis** .................... 109
   *James Foshee, Alfred Marc Iloreta*
   *Gurston G Nyquist, Marc R Rosen*
   - Epidemiology  *109*
   - Anatomy  *110*
   - Management  *111*
   - Anterior Epistaxis  *112*
   - Posterior Epistaxis  *117*

## 7. Common Nasal and Sinus Pathologies in Children 125
*Karin PQ Oomen, Ashutosh Kacker*
- Sinusitis  *125*
- Epistaxis  *128*

*Index*  *131*

# Anatomy and Physiology of the Nose, Paranasal Sinuses, and Olfaction

*Chapter 1*

*Angela Donaldson, Roheen Raithatha*

## ANATOMY OF THE OLFACTORY SYSTEM

### Introduction

It is estimated that approximately 1–2% of the population suffers from disorders of taste and smell.[1] There are several categories of olfactory dysfunction including anosmia, hyposmia and dysosmia. Anosmia is the total loss of ability to detect odorants while hyposmia is the decreased ability to detect such odors. Dysosmia has two types, referred to as phantosmia and parosmia. Phantosmia is characterized as the perception of an odorant being present when it is not, whereas parosmia is the perception of an altered sense of smell. Patients with dysosmia tend to perceive malodorous smells such as rotten fumes and gas leaks.

### Olfactory Anatomy

#### Nasal Passage

Olfaction is determined primarily by the ability of odorants to reach the olfactory epithelium at the roof of the nasal cavity. This action occurs through inhalation into the nasal cavity and through retronasal flow from the nasopharynx and oropharynx. Based on a large scale model study, there is evidence that 50% of the total airflow goes through the middle turbinate but only 15% of airflow reaches the olfactory region.[2]

#### Olfactory Mucus

Once the odorants have traversed the nasal passageway, they must interact with the olfactory mucus which covers the olfactory epithelium. Odorants are classified based on their solubility, but this is not the only variable in reaching the olfactory receptors. The composition of the mucus also determines the transit time to the receptors, and adrenergic, cholinergic and peptidergic agents are known to affect the thickness of the mucus layer.

## Olfactory Epithelium

The olfactory epithelium is located approximately 7 cm into the nasal cavity, where it spans around 1 cm² on each side of midline. It is found in the cribriform plate, upper septum, and the medial portion of the middle and superior turbinates. On nasal endoscopy, it appears as thick pale mucosa adjacent to pink respiratory epithelium. The olfactory epithelium consists of the olfactory mucosa and lamina propria, which is separated by a basement membrane. The olfactory mucosa contains olfactory receptor neurons (ORNs), sustentacular cells, basal cells, microvillar cells, and the Bowman's gland ducts. The lamina propria contains the Bowman's gland, bundles of olfactory axons, and blood vessels. The ORN is a bipolar neuron which has a club shaped end that projects peripherally and contains immotile cilia. The olfactory receptors which are found on these cilia are the gateway to olfactory transmission. Single non-myelinated axons project toward the olfactory bulb after they have come together to form myelinated fascicles and are referred to as filae olfactoria. These filae olfactoria travel through the foramina of the cribriform plate to reach the olfactory bulb. Sustentacular cells form a tight barrier around the distal dendrite of the ORN and are thought to aid in the removal of odorants after perception and to prevent toxin exposure. The basal cells of the olfactory epithelium include the horizontal and globose cells, which are thought to be the stem cells of the olfactory system. Within the lamina propria, the Bowman's glands produce mucus which travels through ducts in the olfactory mucosa and are secreted onto the olfactory epithelium.

## Olfactory Bulb

The olfactory bulb is located at the base of the frontal cortex in the anterior cranial fossa. The bulb consists of multiple layers including the glomerular layer, olfactory nerve layer, external and internal plexiform layers, mitral and granule cell layers. Olfactory nerve bundles from the ORN from glomeruli that subsequently synapse with second cell neurons (mitral and tufted cell) and intrinsic neurons. From the olfactory bulb, synapses are transmitted to the olfactory cortex. The olfactory cortex has extrinsic connections to other areas of the brain including the lateral hypothalamus and the hippocampus, which may explain why smell often evokes strong memories.[3]

## Olfactory Physiology

The process of olfaction occurs when inhalation of an odorant reaches the olfactory cleft and goes through the olfactory mucus.

From here the odorant must attach to specific olfactory receptors on the cilia of the ORN. This elicits a G protein second messenger pathway which upregulates cyclic adenosine monophosphate (cAMP) leading to depolarization of the cell and firing of action potentials to the olfactory bulb. A decrease in the odor perception is due to adaptation. It is believed that increased intracellular $Ca^{+2}$ ions block cAMP, and therefore plays a vital role in adaptation.[4,5]

## Differential Diagnosis

The most common causes of olfactory disorders are post-upper respiratory infection (URI), head trauma, nasal and sinus disease, toxins, congenital disorders, and idiopathic processes. These etiologies can be separated into conductive and sensorineural disorders.

### Conductive Disorders

Conductive disorders include septal deviation, nasal polyps, sinonasal tumors, nasal and sinus disease, and prior surgery.

Depending on the significance of the septal deviation there may be some obstruction of nasal airflow. Several studies have reported traumatic nasal deformity as a cause for olfactory loss, but none have used objective olfactory testing to confirm this hypothesis. A few studies have looked at the impact of surgery on olfactory disorders and there has not been a meaningful improvement documented in these.[6] Many authors would agree that a severe septal deflection may cause olfactory loss but deformity to this degree is rare.

Nasal polyps may cause obstruction in airflow leading to anosmia or hyposmia. Sinonasal tumors such as inverting papilloma, adenomas, squamous cell carcinomas, and esthesioneuroblastomas may also cause nasal obstruction and hyposmia. However, these lesions commonly cause unilateral olfactory loss and therefore may not be the presenting symptom.

Chronic rhinosinusitis and edema of the nasal mucosa can cause obstruction of airflow to the olfactory cleft. In addition to obstruction, a study by Kern in 2004 showed evidence of apoptosis of the olfactory epithelium due to chronic sinusitis and persistent swelling.[7]

Prior surgeries including total laryngectomy and tracheostomy divert airflow away from the nasal cavity, and therefore lead to a decreased sense of smell.

### Sensorineural Disorders

Sensorineural disorders include post-URI, trauma, congenital disorders and aging.

Typically olfactory loss due to a URI recovers within a few days of illness; however, a small subset of these patients never recovers normal olfactory function. The incidence of this is much higher in women and the elderly population. Thirty-two to sixty-seven percent of patients regain a significant amount of function, which can take anywhere from a couple of weeks to several years after the illness has resolved.[8] Unfortunately, less than 10% of those patients who experience persistent olfactory loss after a URI will return to absolutely normal function.

The incidence of olfactory loss after trauma is between 5% and 10%. Head trauma is more likely to result in total anosmia when compared to URI etiology. The loss of olfaction in head trauma is likely due to shearing effect of the axons by the cribriform plate.[9] Blunt trauma to the forehead or occiput is more likely to lead to anosmia, with occipital trauma being five times more likely to result in complete loss.[10]

Congenital disorders account for about 3% of anosmia patients. This is typically an isolated finding seen in the preteen and adolescent age group. The pathology of congenital disorders shows a degeneration or atrophy of the olfactory epithelium or bulb. The most common congenital disorder is Kallmann syndrome. This syndrome is characterized as an autosomal dominant or X-linked syndrome with agenesis of the olfactory bulb and hypogonadotropic hypogonadism.

Aging has long been known to affect olfactory function. As we age, functional olfactory epithelium is replaced with respiratory epithelium. By age 65, 20% of the patient population has olfactory dysfunction, and this increases to 50% by age 80. Alzheimer's and Parkinson's disease have been associated with olfactory dysfunction. In fact, recent studies have shown that olfactory loss is an early sign for both disease processes, even when the patient is otherwise asymptomatic.

Other causes of sensorineural disorders include toxins, medications and HIV. Tobacco smoke is associated with hyposmia in active smokers; however, once smoking cessation occurs, olfactory status returns to baseline. Well debated in the literature, zinc gluconate has been associated with loss of smell after URI. Additionally, HIV has been associated with olfactory loss which does not correlate with disease progression.

## Workup

The most important part of the workup is a detailed medical history and physical examination. Key portions of the history that should be elicited include timing of onset, severity, and symptoms around the time of onset, including URI or trauma. A thorough review of symptoms and past medical history is also warranted. A history of hypothyroidism, neurodegenerative disorder in the patient or their family, and the use of certain medications may endorse a more systemic cause for the disorder. Physical examination should focus on the nasal endoscopy, cranial nerve (CN) examination, and oral cavity examination. Typically, an identification test should be performed in the office to objectively evaluate the severity of the olfactory loss. The University of Pennsylvania Smell Identification Test (UPSIT) is frequently used in clinical situations. This is a 40 question scratch and sniff identification test with a score greater than five, but less than 20, representing anosmia. Other testing such as blood work and imaging may also be warranted. If the patient has an anatomic deformity or obstruction, a history of sinonasal disease, or a diagnosis that is not clear based on history and physical, then a CT scan of the sinuses is appropriate. Images in the coronal section are most helpful as they identify sinus disease in the ethmoid region, tumors, and bony deformities leading to obstruction. A magnetic resonance imaging is useful for viewing soft tissue and potential olfactory bulb abnormalities. Patients who come in with a complaint of taste dysfunction along with a decreased sense of smell should be asked about their ability to taste sweet, sour, bitter and salty. If the patient is able to decipher these flavors, it is unlikely that they have a problem with taste and their symptoms are most likely secondary to an olfactory dysfunction.

## Management

The management of olfactory disorders depends primarily on the cause. Medical treatments including nasal and oral steroids are used to treat nasal and sinus disease such as chronic rhinosinusitis, nasal polyps and nasal edema. Antihistamines and antibiotics can also be used in those with allergic rhinitis or chronic or acute sinusitis, respectively. Oral steroids have been quite effective in improving olfactory function when narrowed airflow passages are due to edema and inflammation. This medication is typically tried for 1–2 weeks but cannot be used on a long-term basis because of the potential side effects of persistent use. Surgical options are also a possibility for patients with chronic rhinosinusitis with or without nasal polyps. Surgical correction of a severely deformed nasal septum may improve airflow but has not been found to make a significant difference in olfactory function. Patients with previous nasal surgery including rhinoplasty, resection of intranasal lesions, and skull base tumors may have scarring that limits nasal airflow, in which case surgery may lead to improvement in olfaction. Unfortunately, a significant number of etiologies do not have a proven therapeutic option. Reports of vitamin and mineral supplementation have shown inconsistent results. Vitamin A and zinc are the most studied supplements for olfaction; however, to date, there is no conclusive evidence that either treatment has an impact on smell.[11] Additionally, this improvement is difficult to prove given the possibility of spontaneous recovery of olfaction. A randomized, double blind, crossover study by Henkin et al. showed that zinc is no more effective than placebo in improving olfactory function.[12]

The most important job of the physician is to educate their patients about the condition and give them steps to improve their safety and quality of life. This includes adding color, texture, and spice to the food they consume and counseling them on the importance of functioning smoke detectors and natural gas detectors in the home.[13] Patients are instructed to be vigilant about checking the expiration dates on foods and looking at the appearance of food before cooking. For those patients with dysosmia, this can be significantly disruptive to their lives. Some literature would even suggest that it is even more limiting than those patients who suffer from anosmia or hyposmia. These patients may benefit from the use of gabapentin and clonazepam which has been prescribed for off label use.

## Conclusion

Olfactory dysfunction can have a significant impact on patient quality of life. Many patients suffer with weight loss, depression, and social isolation because they can no longer perceive food, drink, and environmental stimulus in the manner they once did. This condition is especially concerning for patients working in industries where taste and smell are vital to their productivity and safety. There are multiple etiologies for this relatively common disorder; therefore, a detailed history and physical including nasal endoscopy is warranted. Smell identification test along with imaging studies will help narrow the differential diagnosis and provide the best management strategy for this often difficult to treat condition.

## SINONASAL PHYSIOLOGY

### The Nose

The first of many protective features of the sinonasal cavity are the vibrissae, which are the hairs located just within the nasal meatus.

They help to filter large, aerosolized particles from the inspired air. The next tier of sinonasal defense is the nasal valves, which regulate inspired airflow. The external nasal valve is defined by the angle between the medial and lateral crus of the lower lateral cartilage, the columella, and the nasal sill. The internal nasal valve, which is the narrowest portion of the upper airway, is defined by the angle between the caudal edge of the upper lateral cartilage, the nasal septum, and the anterior face of the inferior turbinate. The nasal valves are dynamic and can increase and decrease the amount of nasal airflow to ensure that air is not inspired faster than it can be warmed, humidified and cleaned.

## The Turbinates

Inspired air then reaches the turbinates of the nasal cavity. The superior and middle turbinates are formed from the ethmoid bone, while the inferior turbinate is an independent osseous structure. Most inspired air passes between the inferior and middle turbinates. The turbinates increase the total surface area of the nasal cavity, thus significantly contributing to warming and humidifying inspired air. The shape of the turbinates allows air to move posteriorly toward the nasopharynx while changing the airflow from a laminar to a transitional pattern.

## The Nasal Cycle

In a normal nasal airway, most people experience asymmetric airflow through the nose, with one nasal passage being more patent to airflow and having increased secretions from serous and mucus glands, whereas the other nasal passage is more congested with reduced secretions. This nasal cycle is regulated by neural control and vasomotor input that results in alternating engorgement and constriction of the venous sinusoids within the erectile mucosa of the nasal passage. The nasal cycle alternates every 2–7 hours on average.

## The Sneeze Reflex

The sneeze reflex of the upper airway is analogous to the cough reflex of the lower airway. It protects the upper airway by removing irritants from the nasal cavity. The olfactory nerve (CN I) conveys special olfactory senses while the trigeminal nerve (CN V) conveys thermal, noxious and mechanical stimuli from the nasal cavity. When the offending agent is present in the nose, afferent fibers of CN V are activated. The efferent parasympathetic fibers then stimulate the nasal mucosa to increase secretions. At the same time, the phrenic nerve stimulates the diaphragm to active inspiration. The anterior abdominal wall muscles then contract, generating a powerful exhalation (sometimes up to 100 miles per hour) during a brief Valsalva maneuver, forcing the pressure exhalation through the nasal cavity.[14]

## The Mucosa and Mucociliary Clearance

When airborne pathogens pass through the first lines of sinonasal defense, they become trapped in the mucus layer (made from goblet cells) of the sinonasal mucosa. Mucociliary clearance removes both healthy secretions and pathogens from the sinonasal airway and is the principal mode of defense of the respiratory system, in particular the paranasal sinuses.

The anterior margin of the nasal vestibule is composed of stratified squamous epithelium. Around the area of the nasal valves, the epithelium transitions to pseudostratified columnar ciliated epithelium, which is found throughout the rest of the nasal cavity (except for the olfactory epithelium).

Mucociliary clearance in the maxillary sinus flows in a superomedial direction against gravity, with the help of propulsion of cilia, toward the natural ostium in the superior medial wall. The anterior ethmoid cells direct their mucus toward their individual ostia and then into the middle meatus. The posterior ethmoid cells, on the other hand, direct their mucus toward the superior meatus and eventually into the sphenoethmoidal recess. The sphenoid sinus also drains into the sphenoethmoidal recess. The mucus in the medial portion of the frontal sinus is carried superiorly (away from the natural ostium) and then laterally along the roof of the sinus. The mucus along the floor and inferior portions of the sinus is carried medially toward the natural ostium, where it then drains into the frontal recess and into the ethmoid infundibulum.

The mucociliary flow from the maxillary, anterior ethmoid, and frontal sinuses is carried to the ostiomeatal complex and then to the posterior nasopharynx. The mucociliary flow from the posterior ethmoid and sphenoid sinuses travels posterior toward the posterior nasopharynx. From here, swallowing directs the mucus into the gastrointestinal tract.

## EMBRYOLOGY OF THE NOSE AND PARANASAL SINUSES

The embryo develops separate nasal cavities around the fourth to eighth week of gestation as the frontonasal and maxillary processes join. The ethmoturbinals develop from the lateral nasal wall at the eighth to tenth week of gestation. The first ethmoturbinal has an ascending portion which becomes the agger nasi cell and a descending portion which becomes the uncinate process. The second ethmoturbinal forms the middle turbinate. The space between the first and second ethmoturbinal becomes the middle meatus. The third ethmoturbinal forms the superior turbinate. The fourth and fifth ethmoturbinals form the supreme turbinate (when present). The maxilloturbinal (which is not part of the ethmoid bone) forms the inferior turbinate.

The nasal septum arises from the posterior midline growth of the frontonasal process and midline extensions of the mesoderm from the maxillary processes. The descending septum merges with the fused primary and secondary palatal shelves to create two distinct nasal cavities.

The maxillary sinus develops during the tenth week of gestation from the invagination of the middle meatus. Also during the same time, the uncinate process and the ethmoidal bulla form a narrow groove known as the hiatus semilunaris. The anterior ethmoidal cells appear as invaginations from the upper middle meatus and the posterior ethmoidal cells from invaginations of the floor of the superior meatus, both during the fourteenth week of gestation. Development of the sphenoid sinus begins in the third to fourth month of fetal life with pneumatization beginning around age one and completing growth by age twelve. The frontal sinus is typically not present at birth, becomes present by age four, and continues to aerate and grow until adulthood (Fig. 1).

The ethmoid sinuses are the first set of sinuses to fully develop, followed by the maxillary, sphenoid and frontal sinuses (in that order).[15]

## ANATOMY OF THE NOSE AND PARANASAL SINUSES

### Inferior Turbinate

The inferior turbinate comes off the lateral nasal wall. It is composed of a central bony skeleton covered by a mucosal layer. It articulates with the perpendicular plate of the palatine bone and the nasal surface of the maxilla. Its function is to help regulate nasal airflow and humidification.

### Nasal Septum

The nasal septum separates the right and left nasal cavities and provides structural support for the nose. It is made of cartilage

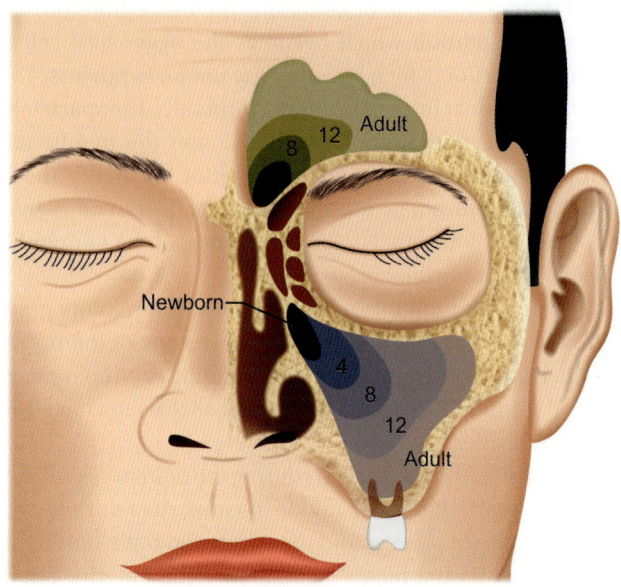

**Fig. 1:** Postnatal development of maxillary and frontal sinus.
From Rhinology: In: David Kennedy, Peter Hwang (Eds). Diseases of the Nose, Sinuses, and Skull Base. Thieme Medical Publishers; 2012.

and bone, which are covered by mucoperichondrium and mucoperiosteum, respectively. The majority of the anterior septum is composed of the quadrangular cartilage. The membranous septum connects the quadrangular cartilage to the columella. The perpendicular plate of the ethmoid bone forms the bony upper one-third and the vomer forms the bony posterior and inferior portion. Finally, the nasal, frontal, maxilla, and palatine bones contribute to the periphery of the septum (Fig. 2).

## Ethmoid Sinus

The ethmoid sinuses are formed from five lamellae: (1) uncinate process, (2) ethmoid bulla, (3) basal lamella of the middle turbinate, (4) lamella of the superior turbinate and (5) supreme turbinate. The basal lamella divides the anterior and posterior ethmoid cells.

### Middle Turbinate

The anterior attachment of the middle turbinate is adjacent to the crista ethmoidalis of the maxilla. The posterior end is attached to the crista ethmoidalis of the perpendicular process of the palatine bone. Superiorly and medially, it attaches to the lateral aspect of

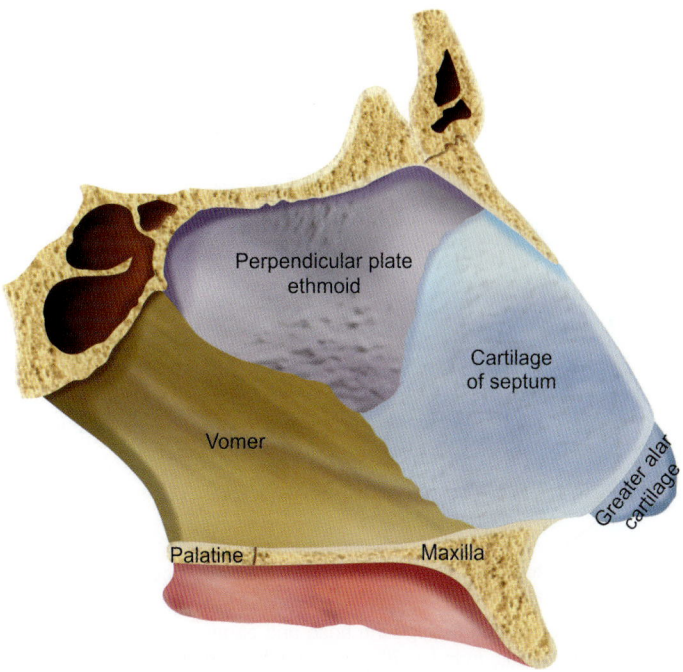

**Fig. 2:** Nasal septum.

the cribriform plate (dividing it into a medial and lateral lamella). The middle third turns laterally across the skull base to the lamina papyracea, where it then turns inferiorly. The vertical portion of the middle turbinate basal lamella is this portion that runs in a coronal plane and attaches to the skull base superiorly and the lamina papyracea laterally (and separates the anterior and posterior ethmoid sinuses). The posterior segment then becomes horizontal. The middle turbinate lies in three planes, thus providing for its stability (Fig. 3).[16]

## Uncinate Process

The uncinate process is a thin, bony structure that attaches to the perpendicular process of the palatine bone and the ethmoid process of the inferior turbinate. Superiorly, it has many possible areas of attachment, including the lamina papyracea and the skull base (Fig. 4). Due to these variations, the frontal sinus outflow tract may drain directly into the superior aspect of the ethmoid infundibulum (less commonly) or into the middle meatus without a direct connection to the superior aspect of the ethmoid infundibulum (more commonly).[17]

**12** *Rhinology Handbook*

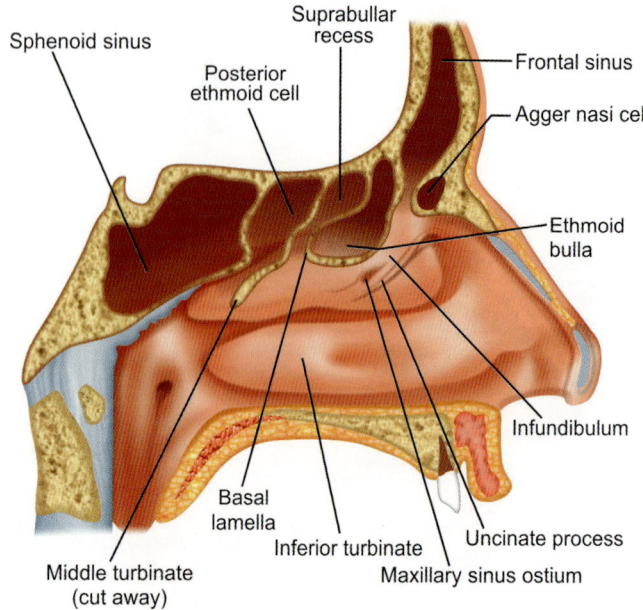

**Fig. 3:** Sagittal section through the nose and paranasal sinuses. The basal lamella of the middle turbinate divides the anterior and posterior ethmoid air cells.

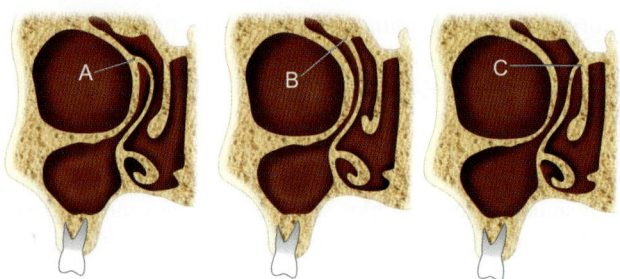

**Figs. 4A to C:** Variants of attachment of the uncinate process. (A) Most commonly, the superior attachment of uncinate process is laterally onto the lamina papyracea. (B) It may attach to the skull base centrally. (C) It may attach to the skull base medially.

## *Agger Nasi*

The agger nasi refers to the remnant of the ascending portion of the first ethmoturbinal. It is the anterior most pneumatized ethmoid air cell and lies immediately anterior and superior to the insertion of the middle turbinate. It lies anterior and inferior to the frontal sinus and forms the anterior border of the frontal sinus outflow tract.

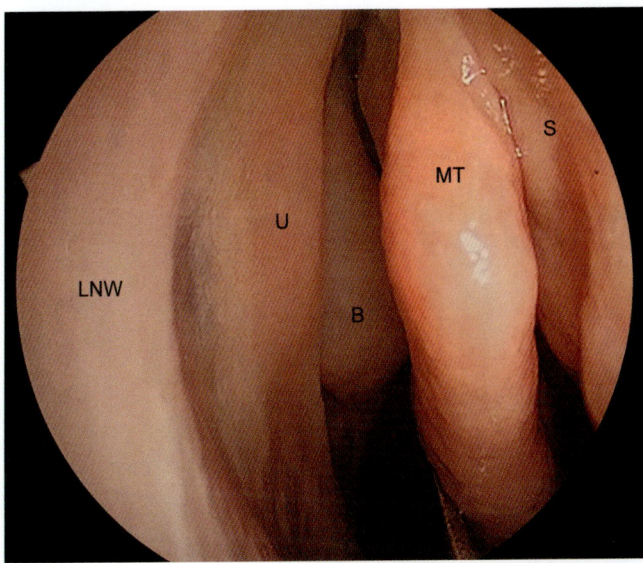

**Fig. 5:** Endoscopic view of right nasal cavity. (LNW: Lateral nasal wall; U: Uncinate process; B: Ethmoid bulla; MT: Middle turbinate; S: Nasal septum.
From David Kennedy, Peter Hwang (Eds). Rhinology: Diseases of the Nose, Sinuses, and Skull Base. Thieme Medical Publishers; 2012).

## *Ethmoid Bulla*

It refers to the largest anterior ethmoid air cell. It forms from pneumatization of the bulla lamella. If it reaches the ethmoid roof, it can form the posterior wall of the frontal recess; however, if it fails to reach the skull base, it results in the formation of a space called the suprabullar recess. It is present medial to the lamina papyracea, posterior to the uncinate process, anterior to the vertical basal lamella of the middle turbinate, and posteroinferior to the frontal recess (Fig. 5).

## *Suprabullar and Retrobullar Recess (Sinus Lateralis)*

The suprabullar recess is the superior space between the ethmoid bulla and the skull base. The retrobullar recess is the posterior space between the ethmoid bulla and the basal lamella of the middle turbinate. The suprabullar recess may extend into the retrobullar recess if the posterior wall of the ethmoid bulla is not in contact with the basal lamella of the middle turbinate. This space is bordered superiorly by the ethmoid roof, laterally by the lamina papyracea, inferiorly by the roof of the ethmoid bulla, and posteriorly by the basal lamella of the middle turbinate.

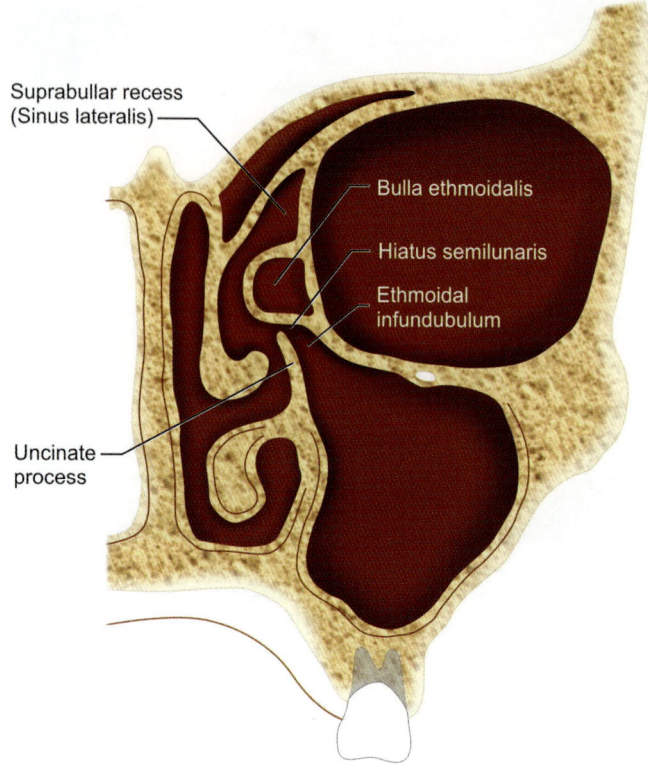

**Fig. 6:** Coronal section at the level of the uncinate process.

## *Hiatus Semilunaris*

It is a two-dimensional opening into the ethmoid infundibulum. It starts inferiorly from a plane between the free posterior margin of the uncinate process and the anterior face of the ethmoid bulla and extends superiorly to the space between the ethmoid bulla and the middle turbinate. The superior hiatus semilunaris is the opening to the retrobullar recess.

## *Infundibulum*

The infundibulum is a funnel-shaped, three-dimensional structure. It is bordered medially by the uncinate process, laterally by the lamina papyracea, anteriorly/superiorly by the frontal process of the maxilla, superiorly/laterally by the lacrimal bone, posteriorly by the ethmoid bulla, and inferiorly by the natural ostium of the maxillary sinus (at its posterior and inferior one-third). It opens into the middle meatus through the inferior hiatus semilunaris (Fig. 6).

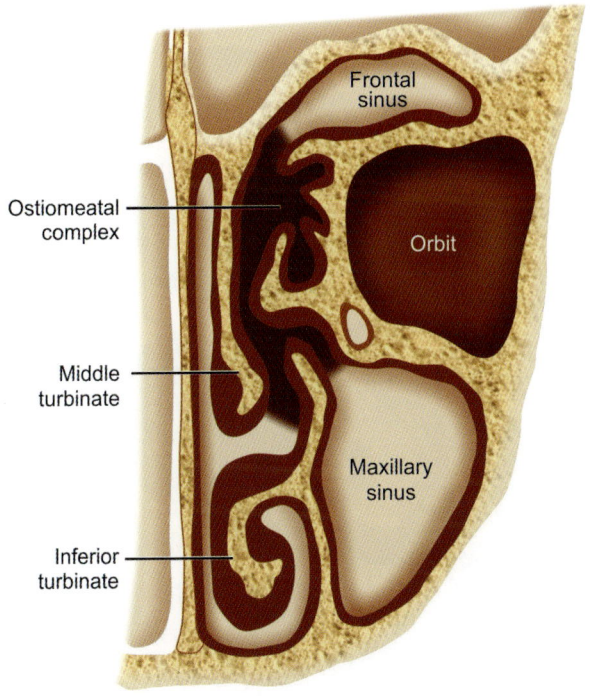

**Fig. 7:** Ostiomeatal complex (in black).

## *Ostiomeatal Complex*

This refers to the conglomerate of structures and sinuses that surround and drain into the middle meatus. It includes the anterior ethmoid, maxillary and frontal sinuses; the uncinate process; and the ethmoid infundibulum (Fig. 7).

## *Haller Cell*

A Haller is also referred to as an infraorbital ethmoid cell as it is present in the floor of the bony orbit, which constitutes the roof of the maxillary sinus. It can cause narrowing of the ethmoid infundibulum or the maxillary sinus ostium. It most commonly pneumatizes from the anterior ethmoid, and less commonly, the posterior ethmoid sinuses (Figs. 8 and 9).

## *Concha Bullosa*

The term concha bullosa is typically used to refer pneumatization of the middle turbinate, although it can apply to the superior turbi-

**16** *Rhinology Handbook*

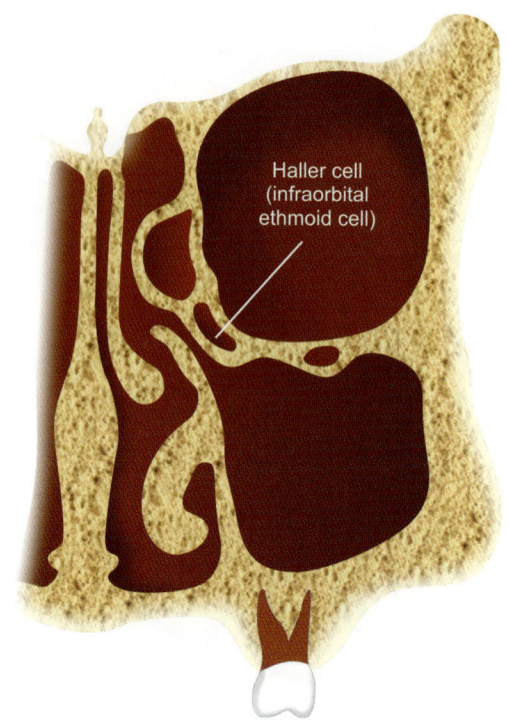

**Fig. 8:** Haller cell.

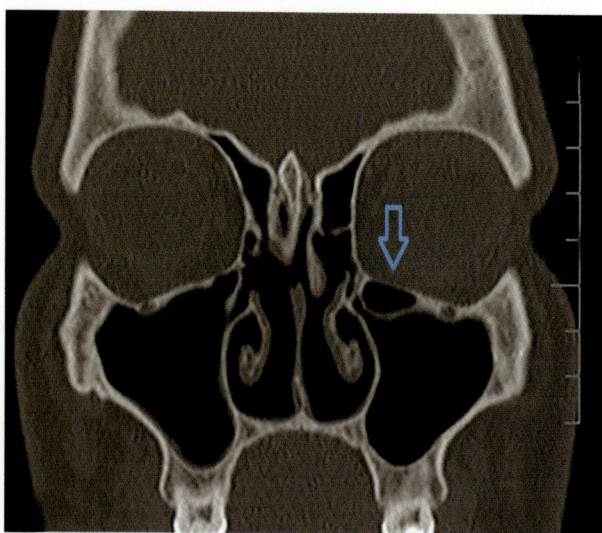

**Fig. 9:** Coronal computed tomography sinuses noncontrast showing a left-sided Haller Cell (arrow).

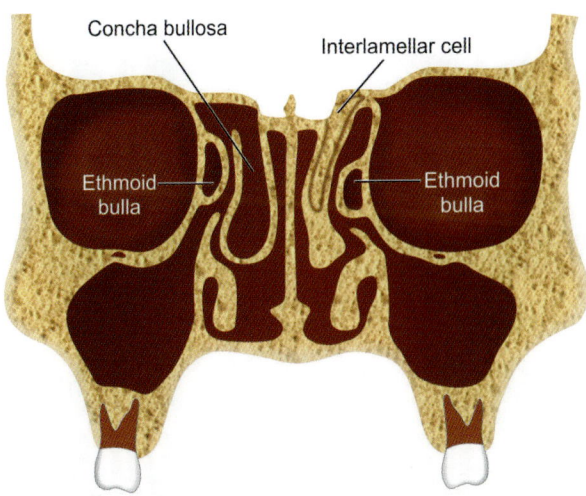

**Fig. 10:** Concha bullosa of right middle turbinate.

nate as well (Fig. 10). The pneumatization typically originates from the frontal recess or the agger nasi. A concha bullosa is a normal anatomic variant; however, it may cause obstruction of the ostiomeatal complex and predispose a patient to sinusitis, in which case surgery may be appropriate. A concha bullosa can sometimes contain a mucocele or a mucopyocele.

## Ethmoid Sinus Roof

The attachment of the middle turbinate to the skull base divides the cribriform plate into a medial and lateral lamella. The fovea ethmoidalis, which is the roof of the ethmoid sinus, is formed by the orbital plate of the frontal bone, laterally, and the lateral lamella of the cribriform plate, medially. The lateral aspect of the ethmoid roof is about 0.5 mm thick, whereas the lateral lamella has a thickness of only 0.2 mm. The thinnest area of the ethmoid roof is present along a groove in the lateral lamella at the site of the anterior ethmoid artery (AEA) (0.05 mm thick) and is the most common site for iatrogenic cerebrospinal fluid (CSF) leak during sinus surgery.

Keros described three configurations of the depth of the olfactory fossa, each of which depends on the length of the lateral lamella of the cribriform plate (Figs. 11A to D). As Keros type increases, there is lesser contribution from the thick frontal bone, with more of the ethmoid roof being formed by the thin lateral lamella. Thus, as Keros type increases, there is an increased risk of CSF leak.

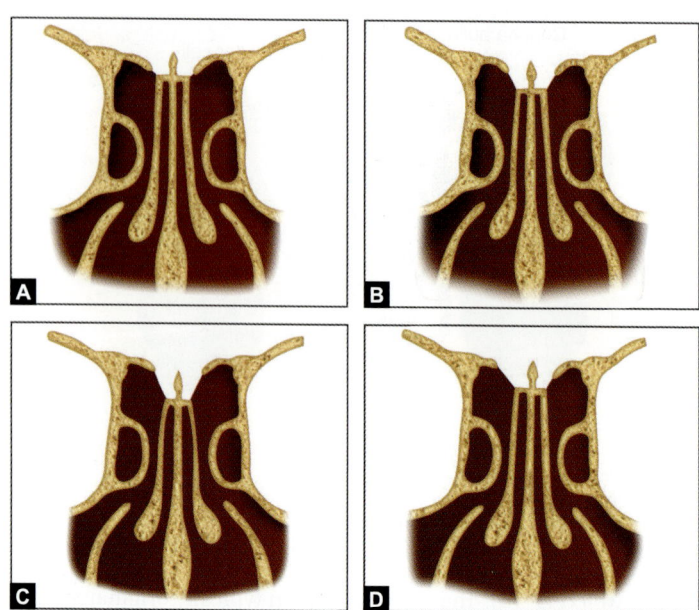

**Figs. 11A to D:** Keros classification. (A) Keros type type 1:1-3 mm; (B) Keros type 2:4-7 mm; (C) Keros type 3:8-16 mm (D) Asymmetric skull base.

*Keros type 1*: The olfactory fossa is 1–3 mm deep, the lateral lamella is short, and the fovea ethmoidalis is at almost the same plane as the cribriform plate.

*Keros type 2*: The olfactory fossa is 4–7 mm deep with a longer lateral lamella.

*Keros type 3*: The olfactory fossa is 8–16 mm deep, and the fovea ethmoidalis lies significantly above the level of the cribriform plate; this configuration leads to the highest risk of injury to the lateral lamella of the cribriform plate due to its steep angle and its thin, overlying bone.

The AEA is an important landmark within the ethmoid skull base. It runs in an anteromedial direction from the orbit to enter the skull base in the lateral lamella of the cribriform plate. The AEA then typically runs along the skull base, although, in well-pneumatized ethmoid sinuses, it may be found 1–3 mm below the roof of the skull base in a mesentery.

## Posterior Ethmoid Sinus

The boundaries of the posterior ethmoid sinus are the basal lamella of the middle turbinate anteriorly, the anterior face of the sphenoid posteriorly, the lamina papyracea laterally, the superior/supreme turbinate medially, and the fovea ethmoidalis superiorly. The posterior ethmoid sinus drains into the superior meatus.

## Superior and Supreme Turbinates

The superior and (if present) supreme turbinates are attached to the lateral nasal wall and the anterior skull base. The superior nasal meatus and supreme nasal meatus lie underneath their respective turbinates. The sphenoethmoidal recess is the space between the superior turbinate laterally, the roof of the nose superiorly, and the nasal septum medially. Its posterior border is the anterior face of the sphenoid sinus.

## Onodi Cell

Also known as a sphenoethmoidal cell, an Onodi cell is a posterior ethmoid cell that is pneumatized far laterally and superiorly to the sphenoid sinus (Fig. 12). The sphenoid sinus lies medially and inferiorly to the most posterior cell of the posterior ethmoid complex. The optic nerve and carotid artery often are found in the lateral wall of the Onodi cell (as opposed to the lateral wall of the sphenoid sinus) and can, sometimes, be exposed.

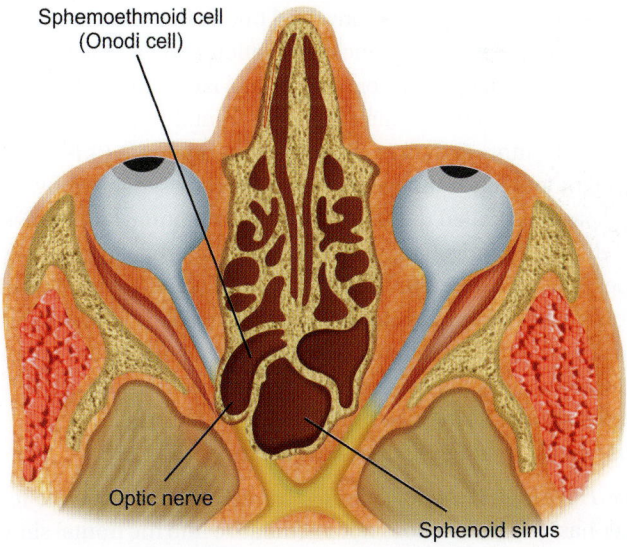

**Fig. 12:** Onodi cell on right side.

## Maxillary Sinus

### Nasal Fontanelles

These are areas of the lateral nasal wall where no bone exists and are found above the insertion of the inferior turbinate. The middle meatus and maxillary sinus are separated only by a layer of periosteum, which can cause the fontanelles to be sites of accessory ostia to the maxillary sinus. The anterior fontanelle is anterior and inferior to the uncinate process while the posterior fontanelle lies posterior and superior.

The natural ostium of the maxillary sinus lies within the posterior one-third of the ethmoid infundibulum. The boundaries of a normal maxillary sinus are as follows: the alveolar portion of the maxilla inferiorly, the zygoma laterally, the floor of the orbit superiorly, the pterygopalatine fossa and infratemporal fossa posteriorly, and the inferior turbinate/uncinate process medially.[18]

## Frontal Sinus

The frontal recess is the most anterior and superior part of the anterior ethmoid complex and communicates with the frontal sinus. The anterior and superior part of the middle turbinate forms the medial wall of the frontal recess while the lamina papyracea forms the lateral wall. It is bounded by the agger nasi cell anteriorly. The recess takes the shape of an inverted funnel in the sagittal section. The frontal recess has significant variation and can be obstructed by a well-pneumatized agger nasi cell or a large ethmoid bulla.

The frontal sinus aerates into the frontal bone. The anterior table (4–12 mm) is thicker than the posterior table (0.1–4.8 mm). The right and left frontal sinuses are typically separated by a thin bony partition called the frontal intersinus septum. Sometimes, an air cell may extend laterally over the superior orbital rim, giving the appearance of a septation in the lateral wall of the frontal sinus. This cell is called a supraorbital ethmoid cell since it is pneumatized from an ethmoid air cell of the orbital plate of the frontal bone. On endoscopic view, the ostium of a supraorbital ethmoid cell is located posterior and lateral to the frontal sinus ostium.

*Four types of frontal cells have been described (Fig. 13):*

*Type 1*: A single anterior ethmoid air cell located superior to the agger nasi cell, which does not pneumatize into the frontal sinus.

*Type 2*: Multiple tiered anterior ethmoid cells superior to the agger nasi cell.

*Anatomy and Physiology of the Nose, Paranasal Sinuses, and Olfaction* 21

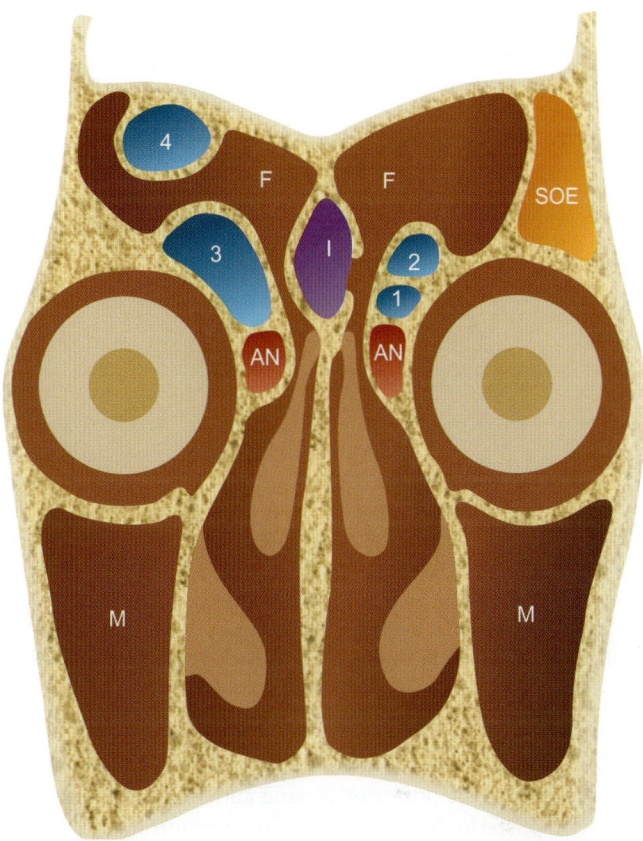

**Fig. 13:** Coronal representation of frontal sinus and recess anatomy.
(M: Maxillary sinus; F: Frontal sinus; AN: Agger nasi cell; 1–4: type 1–4 frontal cells; SOE: Supraorbital ethmoid cell; I: Frontal intersinus septal cell).
From David Kennedy, Peter Hwang (Eds). Rhinology: Diseases of the Nose, Sinuses, and Skull Base. Thieme Medical Publishers; 2012.

*Type 3*: Single large anterior ethmoid cell superior to the agger nasi cell, which extends into the frontal sinus and has a connection to the frontal recess.

*Type 4*: An anterior ethmoid cell that appears to be completely contained within the frontal sinus.

## Sphenoid Sinus

The sphenoid sinus is the most posterior and medially located paranasal sinus and drains into the sphenoethmoidal recess. The natural ostium of the sphenoid sinus is located on the face of the sphenoid sinus itself and is located 7 cm back (at a 30° angle) from

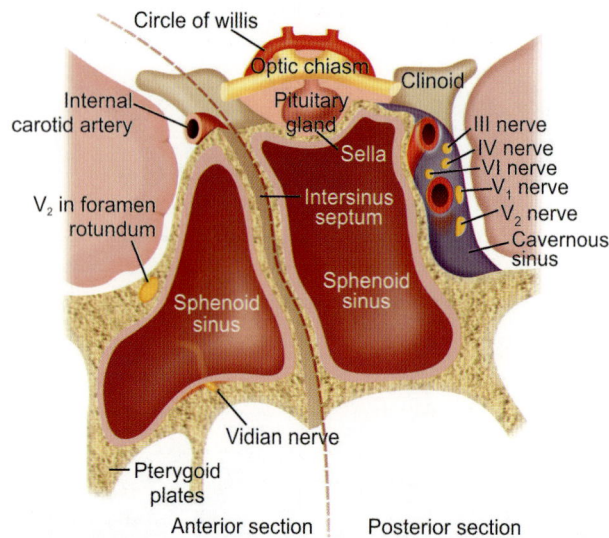

**Fig. 14:** Sphenoid sinus anatomy. The drawing is in an oblique plane, with the left side of the drawing demonstrating structures present more anteriorly, whereas the right side of the drawing shows more posterior structures.
From David Kennedy, Peter Hwang (Eds). Rhinology: Diseases of the Nose, Sinuses, and Skull Base. Thieme Medical Publishers; 2012.

the nasal spine in an adult. The ostium is located 1–1.5 cm above the superior aspect of the posterior choana and lies between the nasal septum and posterior insertion of the superior turbinate.

The roof of the sphenoid sinus is known as the planum sphenoidale. The sella turcica is the bony covering over the pituitary gland and is located in the posterior, superior aspect of the sphenoid sinus. The posterior wall of the sphenoid sinus meets the planum sphenoidale at the tuberculum sellae. The clivus lies just inferior to the sella turcica and is made of thick bone that forms the posterior inferior wall of the sphenoid sinus. The sphenoid rostrum forms the anterior face and floor of the sinus and articulates anteriorly with the vomer of the nasal septum. A sphenoid intersinus septum divides the right and left sphenoid sinuses. It is common for the right and left sphenoid sinuses to develop asymmetrically, and the intersinus septum can be deviated unilaterally with insertion onto vital structures such as the optic nerve or the internal carotid artery.

There are numerous important structures that surround the sphenoid sinus (Fig. 14). The pituitary gland lies posterior and superior in the midline within the sella turcica, just below the optic chiasm. The optic nerve and internal carotid artery can be seen as bony impressions in the lateral wall of the sphenoid sinus (with the optic nerve lying superior to the internal carotid artery). The opticocarotid recess can be seen between the optic nerve and internal carotid artery impressions. The cavernous sinus is located lateral to the lateral wall of the sphenoid sinus with CNs III, IV, V1, V2, VI and the internal carotid artery within it. The vidian nerve is located inferolaterally.

## REFERENCES

1. NIDCD Fact Sheet: Smell Disorder, Publication No. 09-3231. July 2009. Website https://www.nidcd.nih.gov/staticresources/health/smell-taste/SmellDisorders.pdf.
2. Scherer PW, Hahn II, Mozell MM. The biophysics of nasal airflow. Otolaryngol Clin North Am. 1989;22(2):265-78.
3. Engen T. The Perception of Odors. New York: Academic Press; 1982.
4. Hadley K, Orlandi RR, Fong KJ. Basic anatomy and physiology of olfaction and taste. Otolaryngol Clin North Am. 2004;37(6):1115-26.
5. Leopold D, Holbrook E. Physiology of olfaction. Cummings Otolaryngology—Head and Neck Surgery, 5th edition. 2010.; 41.
6. Bramely P. Long-term effects of facial injuries. Proc R Soc Med. 1972;65(10):916-8.
7. Kern RC, Conley DB, Haines GK 3rd, et al. Pathology of the olfactory mucosa: implications for the treatment of olfactory dysfunction. Laryngoscope. 2004;114(2):279-85.
8. O'Brien E, Gurrola J, Leopold D. Olfaction and taste. Rhinology: Disease of the Nose, Sinuses, and Skull Base. Thieme Medical Publishers; 2012; 57-66.
9. Costanzo RM, Miwa T. Posttraumatic olfactory loss. Adv Otorhinolaryngol. 2006;63:99-107.
10. Reiter ER, DiNardo LJ, Costanzo RM. Effects of head injury on olfaction and taste. Otolaryngol Clin North Am. 2004;37(6):1167-84.
11. Reden J, Lill K, Zahnert T, et al. Olfactory function in patients with postinfectious and posttraumatic smell disorders before and after treatment with vitamin A: A double-blind, placebo-controlled, randomized clinical trial. Laryngoscope. 2012;122(9):1906-9.
12. Henkin RI, Aamodt R, Babcock A, et al. Treatment of abnormal chemoreception in human taste and smell. In: Norris DM (Ed). Perception of Behavioral Chemicals. Amsterdam: Elsevier/North-Holland Biomedical Press; 1981.
13. Malaty J, Malaty IA. Smell and taste disorders in primary care. Am Fam Physician. 2013;88(12):852-9.
14. Gudis DA, Woodworth BA, Cohen NA. Sinonasal physiology. In: David Kennedy, Peter Hwang (Eds). Rhinology: Diseases of the Nose, Sinuses, and Skull Base. Thieme Medical Publishers; 2012.
15. Wise SK, Orlandi RR, DelGaudio JM. Sinonasal development and anatomy. In: David Kennedy, Peter Hwang (Eds). Rhinology: Diseases of the Nose, Sinuses, and Skull Base. Thieme Medical Publishers; 2012.

16. Walsh WE, Kern RC. Sinonasal anatomy, function, and evaluation. In: Byron J Bailey, Jonas T Johnson (Eds). Head & Neck Surgery—Otolaryngology, 4th edition. Philadelphia, PA; Lippincott Williams & Wilkins: 2006. p. 307.
17. Stammberger HR, Kennedy DW. Paranasal sinuses: anatomic terminology and nomenclature. Annals of Otology, Rhinology & Laryngology: Supplement, 167. 1995. pp. 7-16.
18. Lang J. Clinical Anatomy of the Nose, Nasal Cavity, and Paranasal Sinuses. Thieme Medical Publishers; 1989.

# Chapter 2

# Acute Rhinosinusitis

*Abtin Tabaee*

## INTRODUCTION

Rhinosinusitis broadly encompasses multiple clinically and pathophysiologically distinct disorders that all share a basic defining feature of inflammatory changes of the nasal cavity and paranasal sinuses. The different subtypes of rhinosinusitis are distinguished based on duration of symptoms, underlying etiology, phenotypic pattern, and host factors. Acute rhinosinusitis is defined as symptomatic inflammation of the nasal cavity and paranasal sinuses, incited by an infectious cause and lasting for a period of time shorter than 30 days.[1] The condition is associated with a high incidence, affecting approximately 20–25 million per year.[2,3] Additionally, the condition is treated by multiple medical disciplines including primary care, emergency room, allergy and otolaryngology practitioners. The most common form of this infection is a viral rhinosinusitis, also termed upper respiratory tract infection (URI). Approximately 0.5–2% of all acute rhinosinusitis events represent bacterial infections.[4,5] Although the majority of therapeutic guidelines target acute bacterial rhinosinusitis (ABRS), a critical aspect of managing patients presenting with acute sinonasal symptoms is distinguishing viral versus bacterial infections. Finally, the clinical presentation of acute rhinosinusitis may mimic other disorders and understanding the differential diagnosis and the role of diagnostic studies is necessary.

## PATHOPHYSIOLOGY

### Microbiology

The pathophysiologic markers of acute rhinosinusitis include obstruction of the paranasal sinus outflow tracts, mucociliary dysfunction, and inflammatory changes of the sinonasal mucosa. The preceding events that result in these changes include local tissue injury by pathogenic organisms and the host inflammatory response. Multiple patient and environmental risk factors may additionally predispose a given patient to sinusitis events. Approximately 98% of acute rhinosinusitis events are viral in nature. Common viral pathogens include rhinovirus, coronavirus, influenza, parainfluenza, adenovirus, and respiratory syncytial virus. Although the majority of these events are self-limited, a small subset will progress to bacterial sinusitis. The factors that impact which viral events are self-limited versus which progress to ABRS are complex and are based on the interplay between tissue injury and host defense mechanisms as well as patient specific risk factors outlined below. The inflammatory changes and disrupted mucociliary function initiated by the viral event allow for a more favorable environment for bacterial invasion which then furthers the dysfunctional cycle.

The most common bacterial pathogens in adults with ABRS are *Streptococcus pneumoniae* followed by *Haemophilus influenzae, Moraxella catarrhalis*.[3,4] Other pathogenic bacteria may be isolated including *Staphylococcus aureus, Streptococcus pyogenes*, gram negative and anaerobic organisms. It is notable that the bacterial etiologies vary depending on patient related factors. For example, a higher incidence of acute infections related to gram negative bacteria are noted in patients with nosocomial infections and patients with cystic fibrosis. Additionally, patients with odontogenic infections have a higher incidence of anaerobic bacteria. Finally, the antimicrobial sensitivity patterns vary based on patient and community factors with increasing rates of and methicillin-resistant *S. aureus* and penicillin resistance in the common organisms causing ABRS.

## Risk Factors

Although ABRS events are most commonly felt to be triggered by a viral URI, other factors may predispose a given patient. These include both host and nonhost factors. Anatomic narrowness of sinonasal outflow tracts may be more susceptible to complete obstruction from a secondary source of inflammation, including a viral URI event. The narrowness may result from anatomic variants including severe nasal septal deviation and aberrant paranasal sinus pneumatization patterns (pneumatized middle turbinate, infraorbital cell, sphenoethmoidal cell, frontal recess cell). However, the high incidence of these same anatomic findings in asymptomatic patients raises questions regarding the true relationship between anatomic variants and the predisposition to sinusitis.[6-8]

The presence of chronic inflammatory changes of the sinonasal mucosa either from allergic rhinitis, nonallergic rhinitis or chronic rhinosinusitis is associated with a higher likelihood of acute sinusitis events. The changes associated with these disorders including mucosal inflammation, ciliary dysfunction, and outflow tract obstruction predispose to acute infection by pathogenic bacteria. Additional host factors associated with a higher incidence of sinusitis events include primary ciliary dyskinesia, cystic fibrosis, dental disease and deficiency of the humoral immune system. Environmental risk factors include exposure to tobacco and environmental pollutants.

## CLINICAL PRESENTATION AND DIAGNOSIS

### Clinical History

The diagnosis of ABRS is typically based on clinical grounds including patient history and examination findings. Adjunctive diagnostic studies are used selectively and are individualized. The common presenting symptoms of acute rhinosinusitis are listed in Table 1. It is notable that these symptoms vary between patients and may evolve during the course of the illness in a given patient. Additionally, these symptoms are nonspecific and may occur in other disease entities including viral rhinosinusitis, allergic rhinitis, nonallergic rhinitis and chronic rhinosinusitis. Therefore, the diagnosis of ABRS is made by a combination of clinical factors including clinical symptoms, examination findings and duration of symptoms. Generally, the symptoms of acute bacterial and viral rhinosinusitis are difficult to distinguish early in the disease course. A presumptive diagnosis of a bacterial infection is suggested by the following: persistence or worsening of symptoms after 7–10 days, initial improvement followed by worsening of symptoms within a 7–10 day period, severe symptoms atypical for a viral URI, a rhinosinusitis related complication.[1,3]

**Table 1:** Symptoms of acute rhinosinusitis.

- Nasal congestion/obstruction
- Mucopurulent nasal discharge
- Postnasal discharge
- Facial pain/pressure
- Headache
- Fatigue/malaise
- Fever
- Maxillary dental pain
- Ear pain
- Hyposmia/anosmia

## Physical Examination and Nasal Endoscopy

A number of physical examination findings are suggestive of ABRS in the correct clinical scenario. Anterior rhinoscopy is ideally performed with a nasal speculum and external light source. ABRS is suggested by edema and erythema of the mucosal surfaces of the nasal cavity including the inferior turbinates. Mucopurulent secretions may additionally be identified. Examination of the oropharynx may reveal diffuse oropharyngeal erythema and mucopurulent secretions draining caudally from the nasopharynx. Palpation of the facial bones may reveal tenderness especially overlying the malar and frontal regions. Palpation of the cervical lymph nodes may reveal enlarged, tender lymph nodes. However, this is nonspecific. Although transillumination of the maxillary antrum has been previously described as a method of detecting opacification, this test lacks both specificity and sensitivity, and therefore has a limited role in clinical practice.

The approach to physical examination varies depending on the medical specialty of the practitioner and availability of equipment. Specifically, inclusion of nasal endoscopy in the evaluation of a patient with suspected rhinosinusitis allows for visualization of the posterior nasal cavity, middle meatus, sphenoethmoid recess and nasopharynx. Endoscopy findings suggestive of rhinosinusitis include mucosal edema, erythema and mucopurulent secretions in the middle meatus and/or sphenoethmoid recess (Figs. 1A and B). Evaluation for other sinonasal pathologies can be performed simultaneously. Finally, endoscopic guided culture of mucopurulent secretions in the middle meatus may allow for identification of the pathogenic species and antimicrobial sensitivity pattern. Endoscopic guided culture has largely replaced antral taps of the maxillary sinus given the similar microbiologic yield of the two studies, and the significantly less invasive nature of middle meatus cultures. A meta-analysis comparing endoscopic guided middle meatus cultures to maxillary sinus taps in patients with ABRS reported a sensitivity of 80.9% and specificity of 90.5% for endoscopic cultures.[9] In settings where nasal endoscopy may not be routinely available including a primary care office, clinical diagnosis of acute rhinosinusitis may be made on the grounds of patient history and examination alone. However, otolaryngology consultation and nasal endoscopy may be indicated selectively in patients with atypical history, concerning clinical findings, unclear diagnosis or failure to improve with medical therapy.

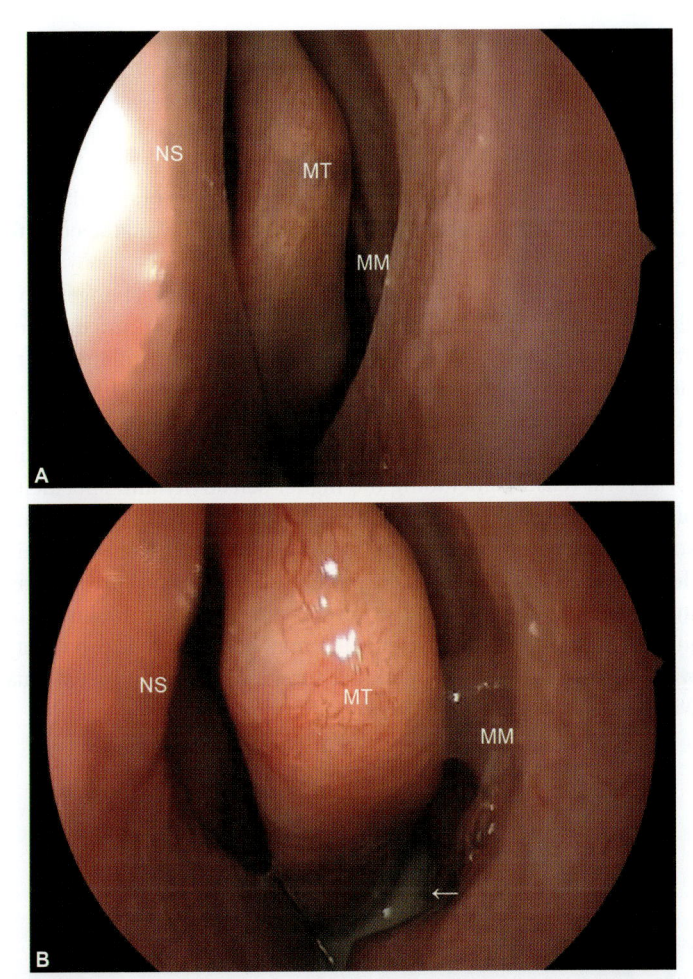

**Figs. 1 A and B:** Nasal endoscopy of a normal left middle meatus (A). Acute rhinosinusitis (B) with diffuse mucosal edema and mucopurulence (arrow) of the left middle meatus. (MT: Middle turbinate; MM: Middle meatus; NS: Nasal septum).

## Radiography

The diagnosis of acute rhinosinusitis is made on clinical grounds in the overwhelming majority of patients. Radiographic studies can not differentiate acute viral from bacterial rhinosinusitis. Additionally, the additional cost and radiation exposure associated with radiographic studies preclude their universal use in diagnosis. Therefore use of radiographic studies is individualized and limited to select situations: a confusing clinical picture requiring additional diagnostic information, clinical concern for complications of rhinosinusitis (intracranial or intraorbital spread), atypical presentation of rhinosinusitis with clinical concern for other processes including neoplasm, severe symptoms concerning for complex sinusitis including severe frontal or sphenoid disease. The last criteria were more prevalent prior to the advent of broad spectrum oral antibiotics when frontal and sphenoid sinusitis were routinely managed with hospitalization and intravenous antibiotics.

The interface between mucosal inflammatory changes and sinonasal bony anatomy is best delineated with computed tomography (CT), making this the study of choice for inflammatory sinusitis. CT findings suggestive of acute rhinosinusitis include opacification, mucosal thickening, air fluid levels and bubbly secretions (Fig. 2). Plain radiographs have largely been replaced by CT scan for several reasons including the higher sensitivity and specificity of CT scan. Additionally, the scenarios in which a radiographic study is indicated are inherently complex and, therefore, highly detailed anatomic images of the paranasal sinuses and surrounding intracranial cavity and orbit structures are necessary. Inclusion of magnetic resonance imaging (MRI) may be indicated in patients with orbital (Fig. 3) or intracranial spread of infection or patients with paranasal sinus neoplasms.

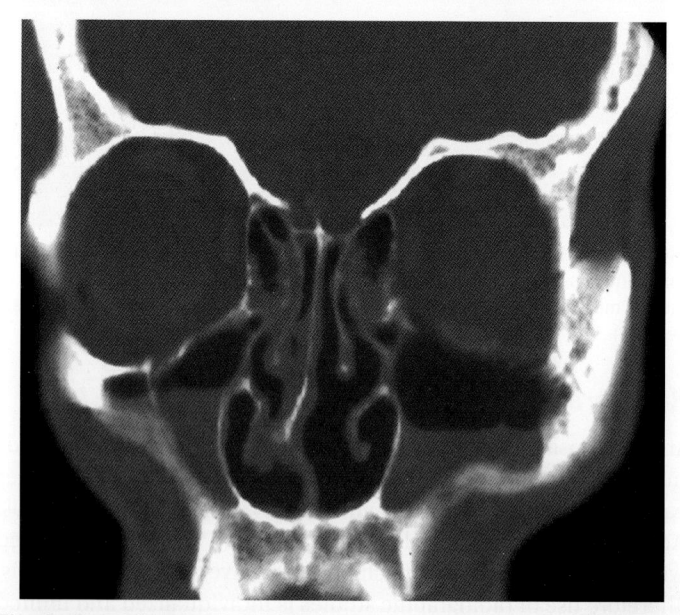

**Fig. 2:** Coronal, noncontrast CT sinus demonstrating bilateral ethmoid and maxillary sinus opacification. Air-fluid levels of the maxillary sinuses are noted.

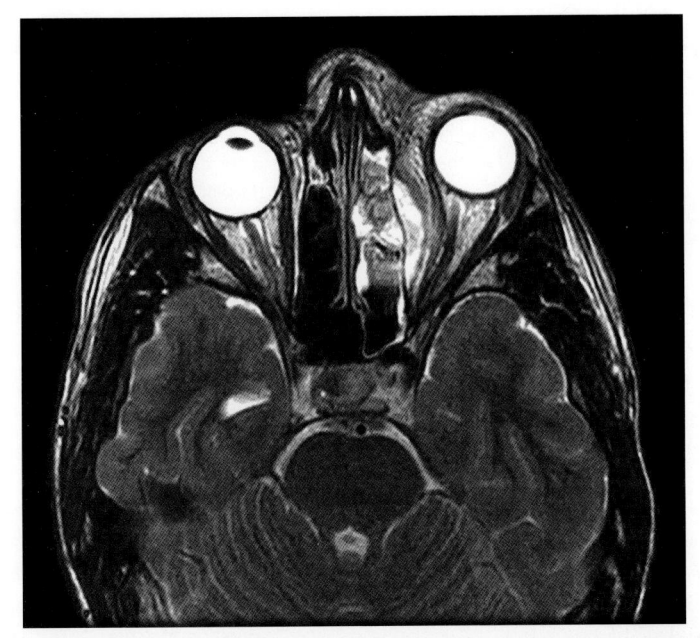

**Fig. 3:** Axial, noncontrast, T2-weighted MRI demonstrating left sided ethmoid inflammatory changes and left subperiosteal orbital abscess with mass effect on the medial rectus and optic nerve. Proptosis of the left orbit is also noted.

## THERAPY

The goals of medical therapy for acute rhinosinusitis are to decrease the severity and duration of symptoms, promote recovery of normal sinonasal physiology and decrease the risk of infectious complications. Treatment strategies for presumed viral rhinosinusitis include expectant observation and supportive therapy. The overwhelming majority of events are self limited. Although the use of symptom directed therapy for viral episodes may help to decrease the severity of symptoms, the impact on the overall duration of symptoms is likely minimal. Available symptomatic therapies for both viral and bacterial rhinosinusitis include topical saline sprays and irrigations, topical and systemic decongestants, mucolytics, antipyretics and analgesics (Table 2).

### Antibiotics

The primary treatment consideration for uncomplicated ABRS relates to the role of antibiotics. The use of symptomatic therapy as described above is similar between viral and bacterial infections, although topical nasal steroid sprays have a greater role in the

**Table 2:** Adjunctive therapies used in viral and bacterial acute rhinosinusitis.

| Therapy (example) | Mechanism of action | Comments |
|---|---|---|
| Systemic decongestants (pseudoephedrine) | Decongestion of sinonasal mucosa (alpha-adrenergic) | Symptomatic benefit. No proven benefit to disease course. Used with caution in patients with poorly controlled hypertension, cardiovascular disease, glaucoma, and prostate hypertrophy. |
| Topical decongestants (oxymetazoline) | Topical mucosal vasoconstriction/decongestion (alpha-adrenergic) | Symptomatic benefit. No proven benefit to disease course. Less systemic absorption than systemic decongestants, potential for rebound vasodilation after 3 days of use (rhinitis medicamentosa). |
| Topical nasal steroid sprays (fluticasone) | Topical anti-inflammatory effect | Multiple studies support use of topical nasal steroids in reducing duration of acute symptoms.[21-23] May be used in conjunction with oral antibiotics. |
| Mucolytics (guaifenesin) | Mucous thinning, theoretically improving clearance of mucous | Symptomatic benefit. No proven benefit to disease course. |
| Antihistamines (loratadine) | Reduction in allergy related inflammation | No proven benefit to disease course for acute rhinosinusitis. May be indicated in patients with coexistent allergic rhinitis. |
| Nasal saline (spray, rinse) | Clearance of mucous, improvement in mucociliary function | Symptomatic benefit. No proven benefit to disease course. Low risk adjunct. |
| Antipyretics/analgesics (acetaminophen, nonsteroidal anti-inflammatory) | Fever reduction, pain relief | Symptomatic benefit. No proven benefit to disease course. |

latter. In patients with suspected ABRS, observation and supportive therapy without antibiotics may be considered as an option since spontaneous resolution may occur in this group. This may be especially appropriate in patients with mild symptoms and can be continued for 1 additional week after the diagnosis of ABRS.

Observation without antibiotics is less appropriate in patients with severe symptoms, fever, clinical concern for possible complications and patients with poor overall health.

Multiple options exist for empiric antibiotics. Selecting an antibiotic is based on a number of factors including evidence based guidelines, local resistance patterns, clinical history of the patient including prior antibiotic usage, results of middle meatus cultures and patient history of antibiotic allergy/contraindications. Several classes of antibiotics have appropriate antimicrobial coverage for common ABRS pathogens including penicillins (amoxicillin, amoxicillin-clavulanate), cephalosporins (cefuroxime, cefdinir, cefixime), macrolides (clarithromycin), sulfonamide (trimethoprim-sulfamethoxazole), tetracycline (doxycycline) and fluoroquinolones (levofloxacin, moxifloxacin, ciprofloxacin). Trials investigating these antibiotics have demonstrated clinical success rates greater than 85%.[1,3,10-16] Interestingly, the results of several meta-analyses support a similar level of success for narrow versus broad spectrum antibiotics in the treatment of ABRS.[11,12,17-20] This coupled with the higher cost, potential for adverse events and antibiotic resistance associated with broad spectrum antibiotics supports the use of amoxicillin as first-line therapy for routine cases of ABRS. Patients with a history of penicillin allergy may be treated with doxycycline, clarithromycin or trimethoprim-sulfamethoxazole as first-line therapy. Use of an antibiotic with a broader spectrum may be indicated in the following situations: moderate-severe disease, resistant organisms identified on middle meatus culture, patients who have received antibiotics in the previous 6 weeks, worsening symptoms after 48–72 hours of first-line therapy, and failure to significantly improve with first-line therapy after a period of 5–7 days. The necessary duration of antibiotics is based on clinical guidelines and individual patient response. The majority of antibiotic trials are based on 10–14 days duration of treatment. Shorter duration of treatment (5–7 days) may be indicated in milder infections and in patients who respond quickly.[1,3,15,16]

## COMPLICATIONS

A number of potential complications may ensue from ABRS. Although the incidence of these events is exceedingly rare in the antibiotic era, the potential morbidity warrants vigilance and appropriate intervention if there are any concerning issues. Intraorbital spread of infection resulting in cellulitis, phlegmon and abscess is suggested by orbital pain, swelling, proptosis, decreased extraocular muscle movement and decreased visual acuity. Radiographic studies (contrast enhanced CT scan, MRI), hospitalization and ophthalmology evaluation are routinely indicated. Therapy is individualized and encompasses adjunctive therapy for sinusitis as above, broad spectrum intravenous therapy and possible drainage procedures in patients with abscesses. The role of emergent sinus surgery, typically in the form of endoscopic surgery of the affected sinuses, is considered throughout the process and may be indicated in patients with orbital abscess, ophthalmologic dysfunction, and in patients with limited orbital infection (i.e. mild cellulitis, phlegmon) who fail to rapidly improve with medical therapy alone.

Intracranial spread may result in meningitis, cerebritis and intracranial abscess. Symptoms suggestive of neurologic, meningitic and systemic toxicity require evaluation including hospitalization, neurology/neurosurgery consultation, intracranial imaging. Lumbar puncture is indicated if there is concern for meningitis. Therapy includes intravenous antibiotic therapy and adjunctive medical therapy for sinusitis. Drainage of intracranial abscess is indicated if there is a significant collection or if there is failure to rapidly improve with medical therapy. The role of emergent sinus surgery is considered in all patients with intracranial infection and especially if there is significant neurologic compromise, intracranial abscess and in patients with milder presentation of meningitis who fail to rapidly improve with medical therapy.

Although not a true complication, one of the most important possible sequelae of acute rhinosinusitis is persistence of the infection and evolution into chronic rhinosinusitis. This is defined as continued symptoms and inflammatory changes on nasal endoscopy and CT scan for a period of time greater than 3 months. The microbiology, inflammatory markers, pathophysiology, clinical behavior and treatment considerations differ considerably between acute and chronic rhinosinusitis, but it is theorized that the initiating event in a significant percentage of chronic rhinosinusitis patients was an acute infection. Although a detailed discussion of chronic rhinosinusitis is beyond the scope of this chapter, it is important to actively monitor and treat an ABRS event until full clinical resolution has been achieved. Persistence of symptoms and inflammatory changes may indicate progression to chronic rhinosinusitis.

Finally, since a number of practitioners are involved in the management and evaluation of acute sinusitis, it is important to identify clinical situations that warrant referral to an otolaryngology specialist (Table 3). Failure to proceed with timely evaluation may cause delays in diagnosis and may negatively impact the disease course.

**Table 3:** Indications for referral to an otolaryngologist.

| Clinical situation | Warning signs |
| --- | --- |
| • Failure to improve with first-line therapy | • Persistent symptoms |
| • Orbital complications | • Orbital symptoms and signs |
| • Intracranial complications | • Intracranial symptoms and signs |
| • Severe sinusitis, especially frontal or sphenoid sinusitis | • Severe symptoms (especially pain and fever), severe signs (toxicity, severe tenderness on palpation) |
| • Recurrent acute rhinosinusitis | • Frequent, recurrent acute rhinosinusitis episodes (approximately greater than 3 episodes per 12 month period) |
| • Chronic rhinosinusitis | • Persistent symptoms for greater than 3 months |
| • Complex host factors | • Immune deficiency, cystic fibrosis, sinusitis risk factors, known history of recurrent acute or chronic rhinosinusitis |
| • Atypical sinonasal symptoms, concerning for atypical process including granulomatous disease/vasculitis, neoplasm, and fungal infection | • Failure to improve with medical therapy, atypical symptoms (bleeding, facial swelling, unilateral symptoms), atypical signs (facial swelling, unilateral process, mass/lesion, and cranial nerve weakness) |

## CONCLUSION

Acute rhinosinusitis is an extremely common condition and encompasses both viral and bacterial etiologies. The diagnosis is typically based on patient history and basic examination of the head and neck. Adjunctive examination tools including nasal endoscopy and radiography (primarily CT scan) are used selectively. Medical therapy consists of supportive care and expectant observation in the majority of patients, including those with possible viral URI and those with suspected mild ABRS. Antibiotic therapy is indicated in patients with persistent symptoms following a 7–10 day period of observation or if there are other concerning clinical factors. Narrow spectrum antibiotics have similar efficacy and are associated with lower cost, favorable tolerability and lower impact on community resistance. Although the majority of acute rhinosinusitis events resolve after appropriate medical therapy, a small subset of patients presenting with acute sinonasal symptoms may ultimately develop complications of ABRS or may have an atypical process. Appropriate and timely intervention is indicated in these patient including otolaryngology referral and possible hospitalization.

# REFERENCES

1. Rosenfeld R. Clinical practice guideline on adult sinusitis. Otolaryngol Head Neck Surg. 2007;137(3):365-77.
2. Schappert SM. Ambulatory care visits to physician offices, hospital outpatient departments, and emergency departments: United States, 1996. Vital Health Stat 13. 1998;(134):1-37.
3. Anon JB, Jacobs MR, Poole MD, et al. Antimicrobial treatment guidelines for acute bacterial rhinosinusitis. Otolaryngol Head Neck Surg. 2004;130(1 Suppl):1-45.
4. Gwaltney JM Jr, Sydnor AJ Jr, Sande MA. Etiology and antimicrobial treatment of acute sinusitis. Ann Otol Rhinol Laryngol Suppl. 1981; 90(3 Pt 3):68-71.
5. Gwaltney JM Jr. Acute community-acquired sinusitis. Clin Infect Dis. 1996;23(6):1209-23.
6. Caughey RJ, Jameson MJ, Gross CW, et al. Anatomic risk factors for sinus disease: fact or fiction? Am J Rhinol. 2005;19(4):334-9.
7. Stallman JS, Lobo JN, Som PM. The incidence of concha bullosa and its relationship to nasal septal deviation and paranasal sinus disease. AJNR Am J Neuroradiol. 2004;25(9):1613-8.
8. Alkire BC, Bhattacharyya N. An assessment of sinonasal anatomic variants potentially associated with recurrent acute rhinosinusitis. Laryngoscope. 2010;120(3):631-4.
9. Benninger MS, Payne SC, Ferguson BJ, et al. Endoscopically directed middle meatal cultures versus maxillary sinus taps in acute bacterial maxillary rhinosinusitis: a meta-analysis. Otolaryngol Head Neck Surg. 2006;134(1):3-9.
10. Snow V, Mottur-Pilson C, Hickner JM. Principles of appropriate antibiotic use for acute sinusitis in adults. Ann Intern Med. 2001;134(6): 495-7.
11. Williams JW Jr, Aguilar C, Cornell J, et al. Antibiotics for acute maxillary sinusitis. Cochrane Database Syst Rev. 2003;(2):CD000243.
12. de Bock GH, Dekker FW, Stolk J, et al. Antimicrobial treatment in acute maxillary sinusitis: a meta-analysis. J Clin Epidemiol. 1997;50 (8): 881-90.
13. Young J, De Sutter A, Merenstein D, et al. Antibiotics for adults with clinically diagnosed acute rhinosinusitis: a meta-analysis of individual patient data. Lancet. 2008;371(9616):908-14.
14. Rosenfeld RM, Singer M, Jones S. Systematic review of antimicrobial therapy in patients with acute rhinosinusitis. Otolaryngol Head Neck Surg. 2007;137(3 Suppl):S32-45.
15. Slavin RG, Spector SL, Bernstein IL, et al. The diagnosis and management of sinusitis: a practice parameter update. J Allergy Clin Immunol. 2005;116(6 Suppl):S13-47.
16. Chow AW, Benninger MS, Brook I, et al. IDSA clinical practice guideline for acute bacterial rhinosinusitis in children and adults. Clin Infect Dis. 2012;54(8):e72-e112.
17. Piccirillo JF, Mager DE, Frisse ME, et al. Impact of first-line vs second-line antibiotics for the treatment of acute uncomplicated sinusitis. JAMA. 2001;286(15):1849-56.

18. De Ferranti SD, Ioannidis JP, Lau J, et al. Are amoxycillin and folate inhibitors as effective as other antibiotics for acute sinusitis? A meta-analysis. BMJ. 1998;317(7159):632-7.
19. Falagas ME, Giannopoulou KP, Vardakas KZ, et al. Comparison of antibiotics with placebo for treatment of acute sinusitis: a meta-analysis of randomised controlled trials. Lancet Infect Dis .2008;8(9): 543-52.
20. Ahovuo-Saloranta A, Borisenko OV, Kovanen N, et al. Antibiotics for acute maxillary sinusitis. Cochrane Database Syst Rev. 2008(2): CD000243.
21. Dolor RJ, Witsell DL, Hellkamp AS, et al. Comparison of cefuroxime with or without intranasal fluticasone for the treatment of rhinosinusitis. The CAFFS Trial: a randomized controlled trial. JAMA. 2001; 286(24):3097-105.
22. Zalmanovici A, Yaphe J. Intranasal steroids for acute sinusitis. Cochrane Database Syst Rev. 2009;(4):CD005149.
23. Desrosiers M, Evans GA, Keith PK, et al. Canadian clinical practice guidelines for acute and chronic rhinosinusitis. J Otolaryngol Head Neck Surg. 2011;40 Suppl 2:S99-193.

# Chapter 3

# Chronic Rhinosinusitis

*Patrick Stevens, Belachew Tessema, Seth M Brown*

## INTRODUCTION

Chronic rhinosinusitis (CRS) is a disorder of the nasal cavity and sinuses that has a significant effect on both the health of patients and their quality of life.[1,2] A distinction between acute, subacute, chronic and recurrent acute rhinosinusitis should be made. Inflammation or infection of the paranasal sinuses is commonly referred to as sinusitis; however this term has largely been replaced by rhinosinusitis, as inflammation of the nasal cavity is concurrently associated with inflammation of the paranasal sinuses. CRS symptoms consist of nasal obstruction, facial congestion/pressure/fullness, discolored nasal drainage and/or hyposmia/anosmia in the setting of nasal and sinus mucosa inflammation that persists for at least 12 consecutive weeks.[3] Patients with CRS can have periods of sudden worsening symptoms referred to as an acute exacerbation of CRS. These patients will have a return to baseline nasal symptoms following treatment.

## EPIDEMIOLOGY

Chronic rhinosinusitis is one of the most common chronic health problems in the United States, affecting an estimated 14.1% of the adult population.[4] This results in approximately 500,000 paranasal sinus procedures performed each year in the United States.[5] According to the American Academy of Otolaryngology, sinusitis results in 18–22 million US physician office visits annually with an estimated direct healthcare cost upward of $3.4–5 billion per year.[6] The overall prevalence of CRS in the United States is 146 per 1,000 population.[4] Sinusitis is the fifth most common disease treated with antibiotics.[7] CRS is a common disease worldwide, particularly in areas with high levels of air pollution. Damp temperate climates along with higher concentrations of pollens are associated with a higher prevalence of CRS.[8]

## PATHOGENESIS

Chronic rhinosinusitis development is multifactorial and the term actually may refer to a spectrum of diseases arising from various causes that have a similar constellation of symptoms. There has been a change in nomenclature from sinusitis to rhinosinusitis representing a change in the understanding that inflammation of the nasal cavity plays a role in the pathogenesis of sinus infections. Inflammation of the nasal mucosa results in blockage of the normal drainage pathways of the paranasal sinuses resulting in both acute infections as well as leading to chronic inflammation of the sinuses themselves. Environmental factors such as pollution, allergens, viruses, bacteria and molds all play a role in the development of sinonasal inflammation (Flowchart 1).

A separate etiology that may predispose patients to the development of CRS is anatomical abnormalities that prevent proper drainage from sinus ostia. Anatomic variations can result in compromise of the osteomeatal complex which is the common drainage pathway for the frontal, anterior ethmoid and maxillary sinuses located inferolaterally to the middle turbinate. A deviated septum and a septal spur can block the osteomeatal complex resulting in decreased drainage from the paranasal sinuses on that side which leads to chronic inflammation and chronic infection of one or more sinuses (Fig. 1). An air containing middle turbinate, referred to as a concha bullosa, may act in a similar fashion by blocking natural drainage pathways particularly of the maxillary sinus. The osteomeatal complex can be narrowed by various other anatomical abnormalities including a maxillary cell known as a Haller cell, a prominent ethmoidal bulla and pneumatization or inversion of the uncinate process. A prominent agger nasi cell, the anterior most

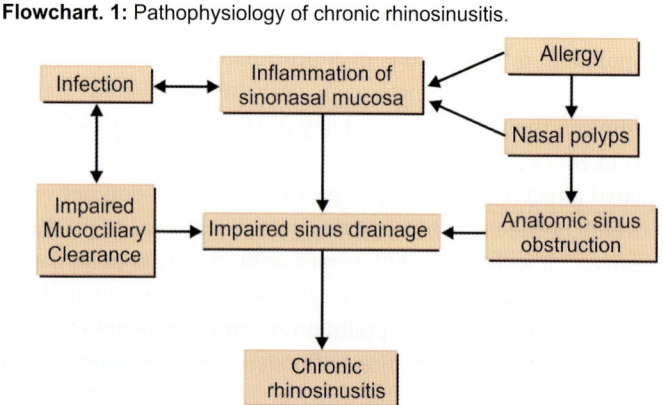

**Flowchart. 1:** Pathophysiology of chronic rhinosinusitis.

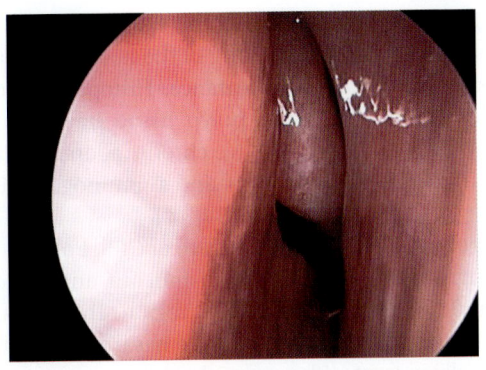

**Fig. 1:** Deviated nasal septum in the left nasal cavity of a patient.

ethmoid cell, can limit drainage from the frontal sinuses in a similar fashion. These anatomic abnormalities in conjunction with mucosal inflammation result in limitation of drainage from the surrounding sinus. Anatomical variations can be diagnosed with nasal endoscopy or computed tomography (CT) in most cases. Patients with these abnormalities will have continued difficulty with the affected sinus and many will ultimately need surgery to correct the underlying anatomy to prevent future sinus infections.

The sinus passages are lined with ciliated respiratory epithelium. Mucociliary clearance is the process by which cilia transport the mucus blanket overlying respiratory mucosa. The mucus of the paranasal sinuses is directed toward the nasal cavity allowing for removal of irritants and microbes. Disease states that compromise normal cilia function result in impaired clearance of infectious pathogens and ultimately recurrent sinopulmonary infections. Cystic fibrosis is an autosomal recessive disorder caused by a single gene mutation resulting in a defective chloride channel (cystic fibrosis transmembrane regulator). The lack of proper chloride transport results in viscous mucus and impaired mucociliary clearance. Primary ciliary dyskinesia, which includes Kartagener syndrome, is an inherited disorder manifesting in severely impaired mucociliary clearance. Upper respiratory tract infections, inflammation and mucosal swelling may also disrupt normal mucus composition, or the mucociliary clearance flow pattern, know as an acquired ciliary dyskinesia. Various pathogens can alter the normal mucociliary clearance system (discussed below).

Allergic rhinitis (nasal allergies) can also play a role in the pathogenesis of CRS and is present in 25–30% of CRS patients.[9] There is an increased prevalence of allergic rhinitis and atopy in patients with CRS, with one recent survey revealing that 56.7% of patients with the diagnosis of CRS also report having allergies.[10] Allergic rhinitis results in increased swelling of the nasal mucosa resulting in impairment of mucociliary clearance. Histopathological studies of ethmoidal tissue and nasal polyp tissue have demonstrated that allergic patients with CRS have chronic allergic inflammation including increased plasma cells and immunoglobulin E (IgE) levels.[11,12]

Nasal polyps are a common feature of CRS. Polyps are inflammatory outgrowths of the sinonasal mucosa and typically arise from the middle meatus and ethmoid region. They usually appear as semitranslucent, pale growths in the nasal cavity. Patients with polyps typically present with perennial nasal congestion, obstruction and anosmia or hyposmia. Often the symptoms worsen with an acute upper respiratory infection. The etiology of nasal polyps is unknown and may be a result of a wide variety of disorders all of which have an effect on mucosal inflammation.[8] Twenty percent of patients with CRS will have nasal polyps.[13] Children and patients with unilateral polyposis often require further workup. In children with nasal polyps, further workup is often indicated to evaluate for cystic fibrosis. Patients with unilateral disease should at the least undergo imaging and often a biopsy to rule out a malignancy or a benign growth such as an inverted papilloma. These conditions can look very similar to polyposis on an exam. Other coexisting disorders which may present with nasal polyposis include: Churg-Strauss syndrome, ciliary dyskinesia and Samter's triad (the constellation of nasal polyps, asthma and aspirin sensitivity). Overall, patients with CRS and nasal polyps should be considered separately from patients without nasal polyposis as treatment regimens may differ (Fig. 2).

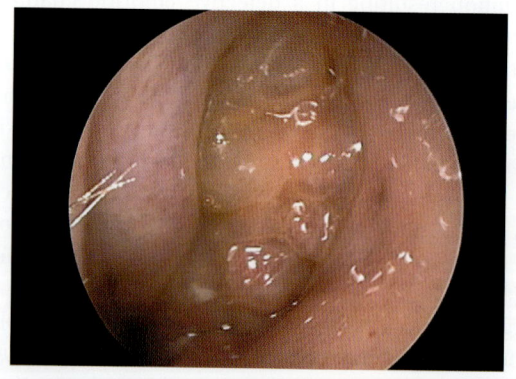

**Fig. 2:** Nasal polyp in left middle meatus of a patient with chronic rhinosinusitis with polyposis.

## CLINICAL PRESENTATION, EVALUATION AND DIAGNOSIS

The symptomatology of patients with CRS varies from patient to patient but includes the following[14] (Table 1):

By definition symptoms must be present for a period of at least 12 weeks to qualify for a diagnosis of CRS. This differentiates CRS from acute (symptoms less than 4 weeks) and subacute (symptoms of 4–12 weeks). While there are numerous similarities between the presentations of acute and CRS, the symptoms of CRS tend to be less severe.

The nasal cavity should be examined using a nasal speculum and a headlight if possible, or at the very least with an otoscope. Assessment should involve examining the floor of the nose as well as the middle meatus for any evidence of purulence or polypoid change to the mucosa. The differential diagnosis includes sinonasal

**Table 1:** Diagnosis of chronic rhinosinusitis.

*Major factors*
- Facial pain, pressure or fullness
- Facial congestion or fullness
- Nasal obstruction or blockage
- Nasal discharge, purulence or discolored postnasal drainage
- Hyposmia or anosmia
- Purulence in the nasal cavity

*Minor factors*
- Headache
- Fever
- Halitosis
- Fatigue
- Dental pain
- Cough
- Ear pain, pressure or fullness

tumors which will require further workup and a tissue diagnosis. Patients should be referred for an otolaryngology evaluation if they present with any of the following symptoms: unilateral only symptoms, bleeding or bloodstained drainage, cacosmia (foul smelling drainage), proptosis, diplopia, epiphora, neurological changes and symptoms refractory to medical management that might require an evaluation for surgical intervention.

In most cases a diagnosis of CRS is made based on symptoms alone; however the American Academy of Otolaryngology-Head and Neck Surgery (AAO-HNS) recommends that a diagnosis of CRS be confirmed with diagnostic evaluation.[14] Nasal endoscopy, CT and allergy and immunological testing are the three main diagnostic tests that are often utilized in evaluating CRS. Purulent mucus, edema of the middle meatus and ethmoid sinuses and the presence of nasal polyps support a diagnosis of CRS. One prospective study found that nasal endoscopy improved the quality of diagnosis and can be used to visualize features such as nasal polyps or discharge (Figs. 3 and 4).[15]

A CT scan without intravenous (IV) contrast is the gold standard for evaluating the paranasal sinuses for evidence of chronic inflammation. Imaging, however, is not necessary for every patient and CT scans should be reserved for patients in the following circumstances.
- Patients who have failed medical therapy—to evaluate for anatomic abnormalities and continued infection/inflammation.
- Rhinosinusitis with suspected orbital or intracranial complication (should be ordered with and without contrast).

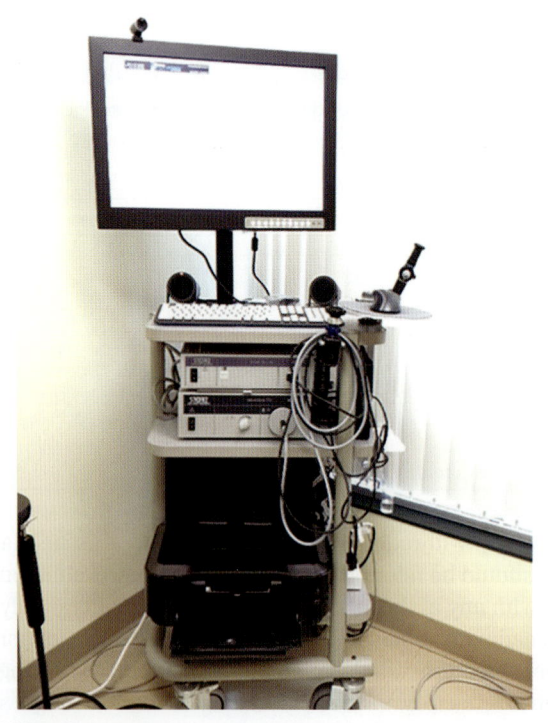

**Fig. 3:** Office video tower.

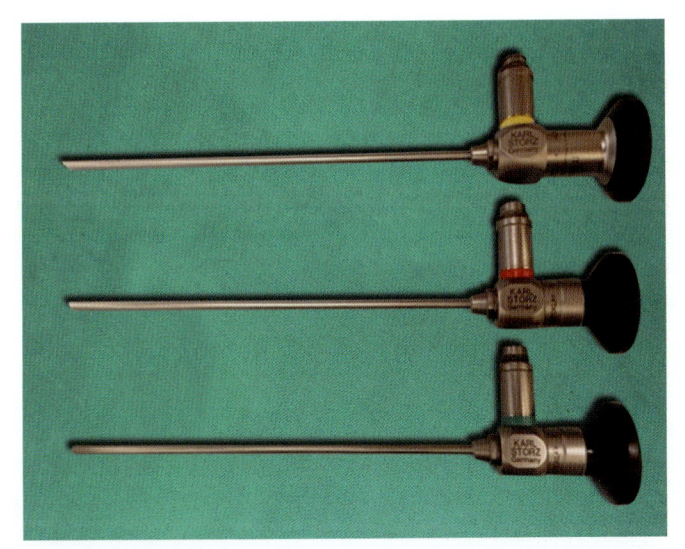

**Fig. 4:** Rigid endoscopes.

- Nasal mass that is suspicious for malignancy (should be ordered with and without contrast).

It should be noted that the severity of symptoms is not often correlated with the radiographic findings on CT.

A diagnosis of CRS requires of two of the following symptoms:
- Endoscopic evidence of mucosal inflammation—purulent mucus or edema in middle meatus or ethmoid region
- Polyps in nasal cavity or middle meatus
- Radiographic evidence of mucosal inflammation

Allergy and/or immunologic studies are indicated for patients who fail to improve or who have symptoms consistent with either seasonal or environmental allergic rhinitis. Allergy testing via skin prick or intradermal injection is adequate. Radioallergosorbent (RAST) testing, an in vitro allergen-specific immunoassay, is a viable alternative to skin testing if the patient has a strong history of anaphylaxis. However, RAST testing is less sensitive relative to skin testing[16] and can become expensive quickly when testing a number of antigens. For patients who continue to fail aggressive medical and surgical management, immunodeficiency may be present. Selective IgA deficiency, common variable immunodeficiency and hypogammaglobulinemia are the most common humoral immunodeficiencies related to CRS. Also HIV should be considered in refractory patients as up to 64% of patients with AIDS will develop CRS.[17]

## SUBTYPES OF RHINOSINUSITIS (TABLE 2)

### Viral

Rhinosinusitis associated with a viral infection is typically self-limiting and symptoms usually last less than 10 days. There is little evidence to show that viral infection leads to ongoing CRS symptoms or mucosal inflammation. Samples of mucosa taken from patients with CRS symptoms undergoing sinus surgery failed to show any respiratory viruses DNA (deoxyribonucleic acid).[18]

### Bacterial

Bacteria are believed to play a role in most cases of CRS.[19] *Staphylococcus aureus*, *Staphylococcus epidermidis*, anaerobic Gram-negative bacilli and aerobic Gram-negative enteric rods are common in CRS.[20,21] Polymicrobial infection is also common in CRS.[22] Bacteria may also contribute to the formation of biofilms adherent to the mucosa. Biofilm presence is correlated with more severe preoperative disease based on radiologic and nasal endoscopic scoring as well as persistent postoperative mucosal inflammation.[23,24]

Common bacterial pathogens such as *Hemophilus influenzae*, *Streptococcus pneumoniae*, *Staphylococcus aureus*, and *Pseudomonas aeruginosa* produce specific toxins to impair ciliary motion and coordination.[1,25] In particular, *Staphylococcus aureus* frequently colonizes the nostrils. In patients with CRS with nasal polyposis, *Staphylococcus aureus* rates can be as high as 67%.[26] Enteroxins secreted by certain *Staphylococcus aureus*, known as superantigens activate T cells, eosinophils and B cells resulting in a cytokine storm locally in the tissue and generating a strong inflammatory response.[27,28]

**Table 2:** Subtypes of chronic rhinosinusitis (CRS).

| | |
|---|---|
| Viral | Typically acute, can exacerbate CRS |
| Recurrent acute | Episodic acute sinusitis with periods of no symptoms between episodes |
| Bacterial | Multiple pathogens, can lead to biofilm formation |
| With polyposis | Allergic patients, aspirin exacerbated respiratory disease, cystic fibrosis |
| Noninvasive fungal | Allergic fungal rhinosinusitis, sinus fungal ball, saprophytic fungal infestation |
| Invasive fungal | Invasive fungal hyphae and necrotic tissue with minimal inflammatory response |

## Fungal

Fungal sinusitis can be divided into noninvasive and invasive. Allergic fungal sinusitis is a noninvasive fungal infection of the sinus with evidence of an IgE-mediated allergy to fungus. Persistent opacification of one or more sinus despite extensive medical therapy is common. CT findings include a rim of hypodensity with hyperdense central material. Allergic skin testing or in vitro immunoassays will usually show an allergy to more than one type of fungus. The disease process is typically unilateral and can result in dramatic bony expansion of the paranasal sinuses or erosion of the surrounding bone of the orbit or skull base. There tends to be a high association in atopic patients. Establishing a diagnosis almost always requires surgery to confirm the presence of allergic mucin (Charcot-Leyden crystals), which is thick, inspissated and light tan to brown to dark green in color. The presence of fungi and degranulating eosinophils should be seen in staining and pathology. Dematiaceous fungi (alternaria, bipolaris, curvularia, cladosporium and drechslera) are typically the offending pathogen. Treatment of allergic fungal sinusitis is initially surgical but the use of steroids tends to help control the disease.

Various terms have been used to describe the sinus fungus ball including mycetoma, aspergilloma, and chronic noninvasive granuloma. The disease is defined as the presence of noninvasive accumulation of dense fungal concretion in sinus cavities.[29] Typically it is an aspergillus infection of an isolated paranasal sinus in an immunocompetent patient. There is no invasion of surrounding mucosa. Patients may present with pain over the involved sinus. The only efficacious treatment is surgical removal.

Acute invasive fungal sinusitis, also referred to as acute fulminant fungal rhinosinusitis, is a fungal infection that invades the sinonasal mucosa. Patients typically are immunocompromised with uncontrolled diabetes, HIV, current chemotherapy or transplant patients on immunosuppressants. Symptoms include a painless nasal ulcer or eschar, periorbital or facial swelling and ophthalmoplegia. The fungal infection does not limit itself at the mucosa but can spread to the surrounding bone and soft tissues resulting in thrombosis of surrounding vessels and necrotic tissue. The time course is sudden with rapid progression and can spread to surrounding structures including the eye or brain. Although multiple organisms can be responsible, mucormycoses or aspergillus are most common. An otolaryngologist should be involved with diagnosis for any patient with suspected acute invasive fungal sinusitis to endoscopically examine the patient and biopsy any suspicious areas.[30] Treatment is aggressive surgical debridement, systemic antifungals but most importantly a correction of the underlying immunosuppressed state. Overall, invasive fungal sinusitis has a poor prognosis and reversing the underlying immunodeficiency is of the utmost importance.

## MANAGEMENT

The medical management of CRS can be confusing due to the spectrum of disease and multiple underlying host and environmental factors. A clinician should base medical management based on the individual patient's symptoms and underlying etiology (Table 3).

## Corticosteroids

Both topical and systemic steroids are used in the treatment of CRS. They function to reduce mucosal eosinophil chemotaxis and increase eosinophil apoptosis. Corticosteroids also decrease white blood cell migration, production of inflammatory mediators, antibody production, histamine release and swelling through a variety of mechanisms.[31] One of the first-line treatments of CRS is topical nasal steroids. Long-term treatment with topical nasal steroid sprays has been shown to reduce sinus and nasal inflammation and improve symptoms associated with CRS.[32,33] Several studies have demonstrated benefit with small to medium sized polyps and for rhinitis symptoms.[34,35] There is a minimal side effect profile associated with the daily use of topical steroid sprays.[36]

**Table 3:** Management options for chronic rhinosinusitis.

| | |
|---|---|
| Nasal saline irrigation | Mechanical washing of sinonasal cavities |
| Nasal decongestants | Reduces nasal mucosa bulk, can temporarily alleviate obstruction |
| Topical steroid nasal sprays | Delivers topical steroids without systemic effects. Can reduce reaction to allergens and decrease polyposis |
| Antihistamines | Reduces inflammation secondary to allergens |
| Immunotherapy | Reduces inflammation secondary to allergens and can decrease need for antihistamines and topical steroids |
| Antibiotics | Decreases bacterial load and maximizes anti-inflammatory treatments. Should be culture driven when possible |
| Oral steroids | Decrease sinonasal inflammation. Reduces polyp size and load |
| Endoscopic sinus surgery | Reserved for anatomical obstruction and cases that are refractory to medical management |

Oral steroids are effective in reducing nasal polyposis and treating allergic rhinitis.[37,38] Acting in the same fashion as topical steroids they are typically more efficacious however have an increased side effect profile, thus long-term systemic steroid treatment is seldom employed. A tapered dose of oral steroids is reserved most commonly for an acute exacerbation of symptoms of CRS and in patients with nasal polyposis.

## Nasal Saline Irrigation

Nasal saline irrigation has been thoroughly reviewed as a supplement therapy for CRS.[39] It has been shown to improve endoscopic findings and quality of life as well as an overall improvement of symptoms.[40] It works by mechanically removing irritants and mucus from the sinonasal cavity thereby reducing inflammation, increasing mucociliary clearance and ultimately decreasing the swelling of the sinonasal mucosa. Isotonic saline rinses tend to be the most popular, however, hypertonic saline solutions have been shown to improve mucociliary clearance in patients with CRS as well.[41]

Contamination of nasal saline irrigation delivery devices might perpetuate CRS. Care must be taken to explain the importance to patients of rigorously cleaning these devices between uses in conjunction with the use of distilled water. Nasal saline irrigation devices should be disposed of at regular intervals as a prospective study showed 97% contamination of irrigation bottles by 4 weeks' time[42] (Figs. 5A and B).

## Decongestants

Decongestants cause vasoconstriction of nasal vasculature through activation of sympathetic nerves causing the quick relief of nasal congestion. They are either administered as a nasal spray or a pill as an oral decongestant. There are no studies to date which have demonstrated quicker resolution of sinusitis. Topical decongestants are associated with rebound nasal congestion and rhinitis medicamentosa and should not be used continuously for more than three days.

## Antibiotics

Antibiotic therapy should provide broad-spectrum coverage to include the organisms discussed above. Antibiotics reduce bacterial load or treat acute bacterial infections in CRS patients. However, bacteria cultured from patients with CRS demonstrate increased

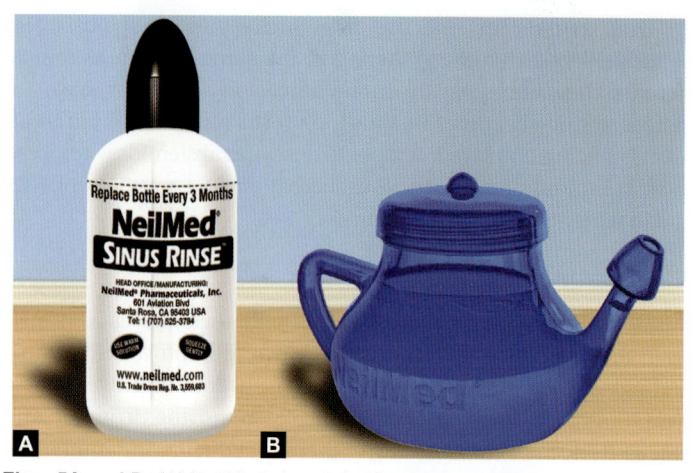

**Figs. 5A and B:** (A) NeilMed sinus irrigation bottle and (B) Neti pot

antibiotic resistance. Commonly used agents include amoxicillin, amoxicillin-clavulanate, clindamycin, sulfamethoxazole/trimethoprim and levofloxacin. The role of antibiotics in CRS is to return symptoms to baseline during an acute exacerbation.[43] Antibiotics are typically used for 3–4 weeks to decrease bacterial load and maximize the anti-inflammatory effect.[44] Culture driven antibiotic therapy can be employed in patients with CRS to narrow the spectrum of treatment and to localize the offending bacteria. This is also important as there has been an increasing predominance of methicillin-resistant *Staphylococcus aureus* in community acquired rhinosinusitis. A meta-analysis reviewing endoscopic middle meatal cultures found results similar to maxillary sinus aspirates.[45] This is a relatively easy procedure, done in the otolaryngologist's office that can assist in guiding antibiotic selection.

## Antihistamines and Immunotherapy

Allergy treatments are helpful for patients with allergic rhinitis and CRS as it will reduce mucosal inflammation. Oral antihistamines are first-line treatment for atopic patients. Allergy testing is usually recommended in patients with chronic nasal congestion refractory to medical management. Immunotherapy may be useful in decreasing allergic rhinitis symptoms ultimately decreasing CRS symptoms.

## Surgical Intervention

Surgical therapy is reserved for a small percentage of patients with CRS. These are patients who fail medical management or have imaging that supports anatomic abnormalities that are amenable to surgical intervention. Patients with massive polyposis rarely respond to medical treatment and surgery will relieve symptoms and allow for the establishment of drainage pathways. Topical steroids are typically used following surgical removal of nasal polyps; however, the recurrence rate of polyposis is high. Other surgical indications include suspected fungal rhinosinusitis, concern for malignancy and mucocele formation.

## COMPLICATIONS OF RHINOSINUSITIS

If left untreated rhinosinusitis may cause local complications. The close proximity of the orbit and the thin bone of the lamina papyracea can allow for spread of infection into the orbit. While grouped into specific categories in Chandler's classification, spread of infection should be thought of as a continuum through which the infection spreads from the paranasal sinus into the contents of the orbit and beyond.

### Chandler's Classification (Table 4)

- *Preseptal cellulitis*—inflammatory edema, no limitation of extraocular movements (EOMs). Treatment involves outpatient antibiotics, topical decongestants, saline irrigation with close follow-up
- *Orbital cellulitis*—chemosis, impairment of EOM, proptosis, possible visual impairment. Patients require hospital admission with IV antibiotics, topical decongestants, and ophthalmology consultation to evaluate vision.
- *Subperiosteal abscess*—pus collection between medial periorbita and bone, chemosis, exophthalmos, EOM impaired, visual

**Table 4:** Chandler's criteria.

| | |
|---|---|
| • Preseptal cellulitis | • PO antibiotics, topical decongestants, saline irrigation, close follow-up |
| • Orbital cellulitis | • IV antibiotics, topical decongestants, ophthalmology consult |
| • Subperiosteal abscess | • IV antibiotics, if no improvement or change in vision surgical drainage |
| • Orbital abscess | • Surgical drainage and IV antibiotics |
| • Cavernous sinus thrombosis | • Surgical drainage and IV antibiotics |

(PO: Oral; IV: Intravenous).

impairment worsening. Therapy includes IV antibiotics, ophthalmology consultation, decongestants, and surgical treatment if no improvement of symptoms after 48 hours, or SPA more than 10 mm or marked orbital signs.
- *Orbital abscess*—pus collection in orbital tissue; complete ophthalmoplegia with severe visual impairment. Treatment is surgical drainage with IV antibiotics
- *Cavernous sinus thrombosis*—bilateral ocular symptoms; worsening of all previous symptoms. Treatment is surgical. Endoscopic decompression and external ethmoidectomy via lynch incision are both options for surgical approach.

Intracranial complications are also on a continuum beginning with meningitis and progressing to epidural, subdural and then intraparenchymal brain abscess. Surgical drainage of any intracranial abscess and long term IV antibiotics are necessary.

Bony complications include osteomyelitis and Pott's puffy tumor. Pott's puffy tumor is a subperiosteal abscess of the frontal bone with underlying osteomyelitis and erosion of the anterior bony table. Treatment is IV antibiotics and drainage of the abscess.

## CONCLUSION

Overall, CRS is a complex disease process with many contributing factors. The underlying condition often results in inflammation of the sinus and nasal mucosa. A wide range of therapeutic options exist and therapy should be individualized for each patient based on the pathologic factors and the patient's symptoms. The overall goal of therapy should be to decrease symptoms and improve each patient's quality of life.

## REFERENCES

1. Quintanilla-Dieck L, Litvack JR, Mace JC, et al. Comparison of disease-specific quality-of-life instruments in the assessment of chronic rhinosinusitis. Int Forum Allergy Rhinol. 2012;2(6):437-43.
2. Bezerra TF, Piccirillo JF, Fornazieri MA, et al. Assessment of quality of life after endoscopic sinus surgery for chronic rhinosinusitis. Braz J Otorhinolaryngol. 2012;78(2):96-102.
3. Pearlman AN, Conley DB. Review of current guidelines related to the diagnosis and treatment of rhinosinusitis. Curr Opin Otolaryngol Head Neck Surg. 2008;16(3):226-30.
4. Anand VK. Epidemiology and economic impact of rhinosinusitis. Ann Otol Rhinol Laryngol Suppl. 2004;193:3-5.

5. Owings MF, Kozak LJ. Ambulatory and inpatient procedures in the United States, 1996. Vital Health Stat 13. 1998;(139):1-119.
6. Tarasov AA, Kamanin EI, Kriukov AI, et al. [Acute bacterial rhinosinusitis: current approaches to diagnosis and antibacterial therapy in out patient setting (recommendations of American Academy of otolaryngology, head and neck surgery, American Association of rhinologists, American Academy of ENT allergic diseases, 2000, Clinical consultative Committee for sinusitis in children and adults, 2000, American Academy of pediatrics, 2001, Center of disease and control, USA, 2001)]. Vestn Otorinolaringol. 2003;(2):46-54.
7. Hamilos DL. Chronic rhinosinusitis: epidemiology and medical management. J Allergy Clin Immunol. 2011;128(4):693-707; quiz 708-9.
8. Benninger MS, Ferguson BJ, Hadley JA,et al. Adult chronic rhinosinusitis: definitions, diagnosis, epidemiology, and pathophysiology. Otolaryngol Head Neck Surg. 2003;129(3 Suppl):S1-32.
9. Savolainen S. Allergy in patients with acute maxillary sinusitis. Allergy. 1989;44(2):116-22.
10. Jarvis D, Newson R, Lotvall J, et al. Asthma in adults and its association with chronic rhinosinusitis: the GA2LEN survey in Europe. Allergy. 2012;67(1):91-8.
11. Van Zele T, Claeys S, Gevaert P, et al. Differentiation of chronic sinus diseases by measurement of inflammatory mediators. Allergy. 2006; 61(11):1280-9.
12. Van Zele T, Gevaert P, Holtappels G, et al. Local immunoglobulin production in nasal polyposis is modulated by superantigens. Clin Exp Allergy. 2007;37(12):1840-7.
13. Settipane GA. Epidemiology of nasal polyps. Allergy Asthma Proc. 1996;17(5):231-6.
14. Report of the Rhinosinusitis Task Force Committee Meeting. Alexandria, Virginia, August 17, 1996. Otolaryngol Head Neck Surg. 1997;117(3 Pt 2): S1-68.
15. Bhattacharyya N, Lee LN. Evaluating the diagnosis of chronic rhinosinusitis based on clinical guidelines and endoscopy. Otolaryngol Head Neck Surg. 2010;143(1):147-51.
16. Bernstein IL, Storms WW. Practice parameters for allergy diagnostic testing. Joint Task Force on Practice Parameters for the Diagnosis and Treatment of Asthma. The American Academy of Allergy, Asthma and Immunology and the American College of Allergy, Asthma and Immunology. Ann Allergy Asthma Immunol. 1995;75(6 Pt 2):543-625.
17. Zurlo JJ, Feuerstein IM, Lebovics R, et al. Sinusitis in HIV-1 infection. Am J Med. 1992;93(2):157-62.
18. Wood AJ, Antoszewska H, Fraser J, et al. Is chronic rhinosinusitis caused by persistent respiratory virus infection? Int Forum Allergy Rhinol. 2011;1(2):95-100.
19. Wald ER. Microbiology of acute and chronic sinusitis in children and adults. Am J Med Sci. 1998;316(1):13-20.

20. Bachert C, Zhang N, Patou J, et al. Role of staphylococcal superantigens in upper airway disease. Curr Opin Allergy Clin Immunol. 2008; 8(1):34-8.
21. Nord CE. The role of anaerobic bacteria in recurrent episodes of sinusitis and tonsillitis. Clin Infect Dis. 1995;20(6):1512-24.
22. Brook I. Role of encapsulated anaerobic bacteria in synergistic infections. Crit Rev Microbiol. 1987;14(3):171-93.
23. Singhal D, Psaltis AJ, Foreman A, et al. The impact of biofilms on outcomes after endoscopic sinus surgery. Am J Rhinol Allergy. 2010;24(3):169-74.
24. Hochstim CJ, Masood R, Rice DH. Biofilm and persistent inflammation in endoscopic sinus surgery. Otolaryngol Head Neck Surg. 2010; 143(5):697-8.
25. Antunes MB, Gudis DA, Cohen NA. Epithelium, cilia, and mucus: their importance in chronic rhinosinusitis. Immunol Allergy Clin North Am. 2009;29(4):631-43.
26. Van Zele T, Gevaert P, Watelet JB, et al. Staphylococcus aureus colonization and IgE antibody formation to enterotoxins is increased in nasal polyposis. J Allergy Clin Immunol. 2004;114(4):981-3.
27. Foreman A, Psaltis AJ, Tan LW, et al. Characterization of bacterial and fungal biofilms in chronic rhinosinusitis. Am J Rhinol Allergy. 2009; 23(6):556-61.
28. Krysko O, Holtappels G, Zhang N, et al. Alternatively activated macrophages and impaired phagocytosis of S. aureus in chronic rhinosinusitis. Allergy. 2011;66(3):396-403.
29. Grosjean P, Weber R. Fungus balls of the paranasal sinuses: a review. Eur Arch Otorhinolaryngol. 2007;264(5):461-70.
30. DelGaudio JM, Clemson LA. An early detection protocol for invasive fungal sinusitis in neutropenic patients successfully reduces extent of disease at presentation and long term morbidity. Laryngoscope. 2009;119(1):180-3.
31. Derendorf H, Meltzer EO. Molecular and clinical pharmacology of intranasal corticosteroids: clinical and therapeutic implications. Allergy. 2008;63(10):1292-300.
32. Benninger MS, Anon J, Mabry RL. The medical management of rhinosinusitis. Otolaryngol Head Neck Surg. 1997;117(3 Pt 2):S41-9.
33. Grzincich G, Capra L, Cammarata MG, et al. Effectiveness of intranasal corticosteroids. Acta Biomed. 2004;75(1):22-5.
34. Badia L, Lund V. Topical corticosteroids in nasal polyposis. Drugs. 2001;61(5):573-8.
35. Langrick AF. Comparison of flunisolide and beclomethasone dipropionate in seasonal allergic rhinitis. Curr Med Res Opin. 1984;9(5):290-5.
36. Gillespie MB, Osguthorpe JD. Pharmacologic management of chronic rhinosinusitis, alone or with nasal polyposis. Curr Allergy Asthma Rep. 2004;4(6):478-85.
37. DeMarcantonio MA, Han JK. Systemic therapies in managing sinonasal inflammation. Otolaryngol Clin North Am. 2010;43(3):551-63, ix.

38. Lund VJ. Maximal medical therapy for chronic rhinosinusitis. Otolaryngol Clin North Am. 2005;38(6):1301-10, x.
39. Harvey R, Hannan SA, Badia L, et al. Nasal saline irrigations for the symptoms of chronic rhinosinusitis. Cochrane Database Syst Rev. 2007;(3):CD006394.
40. Rabago D, Pasic T, Zgierska A, et al. The efficacy of hypertonic saline nasal irrigation for chronic sinonasal symptoms. Otolaryngol Head Neck Surg. 2005;133(1):3-8.
41. Talbot AR, Herr TM, Parsons DS. Mucociliary clearance and buffered hypertonic saline solution. Laryngoscope. 1997;107(4):500-3.
42. Welch KC, Cohen MB, Doghramji LL, et al. Clinical correlation between irrigation bottle contamination and clinical outcomes in post-functional endoscopic sinus surgery patients. Am J Rhinol Allergy. 2009; 23(4):401-4.
43. Lanza DC, Kennedy DW. Adult rhinosinusitis defined. Otolaryngol Head Neck Surg. 1997;117(3 Pt 2):S1-7.
44. Suh JD, Kennedy DW. Treatment options for chronic rhinosinusitis. Proc Am Thorac Soc. 2011;8(1):132-40.
45. Dubin MG, Ebert CS, Coffey CS, et al. Concordance of middle meatal swab and maxillary sinus aspirate in acute and chronic sinusitis: a meta-analysis. Am J Rhinol. 2005;19(5):462-70.

# Chapter 4

# Nasal Obstruction

*Qasim Husain, Ashutosh Kacker*

## INTRODUCTION

Nasal obstruction is one of the most common symptoms of nasal pathology. It is concomitantly one of the most difficult to treat due to its multifactorial etiology. It may occur due to anatomical reasons such as nasal polyposis and deviated nasal septum or secondary to rhinitis or sinusitis. Nasal obstruction itself is the sensation of the absence of nasal airflow with inspiration or expiration whether bilateral or unilateral, and is further divided into partial or complete obstruction. Nasal congestion or stuffiness, decreased smell, the need to mouth breathe, the sensations of fullness, pressure, and blockage are often used synonymously with nasal obstruction. While nasal obstruction may be common, it may not be as benign as it may seem. It has been repeatedly associated with a significant decrease in quality of life affecting functioning at work, as well as concentration in school. In addition, symptoms of nasal obstruction are a major financial burden to the US healthcare system with some estimating its cost at 6 billion dollars annually.[1]

## OBJECTIVE NASAL OBSTRUCTION

The symptoms of nasal obstruction or congestion are subjective in nature, and thus there are many instances where physical examination findings are not consistent with the history.[2] Nevertheless, there are objective measures to determine the presence and severity of nasal obstruction.

### Mucosal Inflammation

Mucosal inflammation is the most common cause of nasal obstruction and should be suspected when the history suggests reversible or waxing and waning congestion. On physical examination, confirm the presence of inflammation by evaluating the nasal mucosa before and after decongestant spray. Mucosal inflammation occurs secondary to allergic and nonallergic rhinitis as well as acute and chronic rhinosinusitis.

## Allergic Rhinitis

Allergic rhinitis (AR) is usually mediated by a type I hypersensitivity reaction with excess production of immunoglobulin E (IgE) antibodies and usually presents with sneezing, itching, rhinorrhea and congestion. AR affects nearly 37 million people in the United States alone.[3] Although AR may occur at any age, its incidence is greatest in adolescence where 80% of cases have symptoms before age of 20 years.[4] Twenty percent of AR cases are seasonal, while the remaining are perennial (40%) or mixed (40%). Seasonal AR presents with watery eyes, rhinorrhea, sneezing, and itching of the ears, eyes, nose and throat during certain seasons, while perennial AR presents predominantly with nasal congestion and postnasal drip that are generally constant throughout the year.

*History and physical*: A thorough history and physical are important in the diagnosis of AR and can guide testing. A personal of family history of atopy increases the probability of AR. In addition, symptom exacerbation at night may suggest an allergy to mites or dander. Conjunctivitis, eczema and asthmatic wheezing corroborate a history of atopy, and in children allergic shiners, nasal salute and mouth breathing are key findings on examination. Pale, blue, boggy turbinates with swollen mucosa and nasal congestion are common findings on anterior rhinoscopy.

*Diagnostic studies*: Skin testing or in vitro serum assays of IgE to particular allergens are helpful to establish specific allergic diagnosis when the history is unclear. Skin testing is a relatively inexpensive in-office procedure that can, with great sensitivity, provide the identification of a wider range of allergens in a timely manner. While more expensive, in vitro IgE assays do not place the patient at risk for severe reactions, offer convenience, provide quantitative results, and may be cost effective in the long run. In vitro testing may especially be applicable for those patients unable to fully co-operate in skin testing, namely children. Serum testing based on the timing of symptoms can be an effective approach in this population. Serum testing for weed, grass and tree pollens when seasonal AR is suspected versus testing for dust mite, animal dander, and molds when perennial AR is a possibility.

*Treatment*: The mainstay in treatment of AR is allergen avoidance, which requires allergy testing to identify causative agents. Once sensitivities are recognized, a comprehensive environmental control plan should be developed which is tailored to the patient. Patient and parent education is a key and should focus on low-cost and feasible measures with a plan for follow-up. Pharmacotherapy is usually needed, in addition to allergen avoidance, in order to achieve symptom control. Topical glucocorticoid sprays are more effective than oral antihistamines in improving nasal congestion symptoms, and are considered the most effective maintenance therapy for nasal symptoms.[5-7] Onset of action occurs in a few hours, but in some patients, it may require days or weeks to see symptom improvement. They work to decrease allergic inflammation by altering gene transcription. With the use of newer generation glucocorticoid sprays, systemic absorption is minimal and provides minimal to no suppression of the hypothalamic-pituitary axis, but growth in children should still be monitored.[8-10] Some of the drawbacks to using topical steroids involve local irritation and discomfort in 2–10% of patients. Epistaxis has also been reported with the use of topical nasal glucocorticoid sprays, but is likely attributable to mechanical trauma and are self-limiting. Dosing should begin with the maximal dose for the patient and gradually be decreased at 1-week intervals as symptoms are controlled to the lowest effective dose. Patients with significant symptoms will require chronic daily therapy, but in some patients dosing can be decreased to every other day or even as needed and still retain symptom control.

Antihistamines may be used in the treatment of AR, especially in patients with intermittent or mild episodes, but should generally be avoided in children and patients with chronic symptoms due to their many adverse effects. Antihistamines both systemic and topical provide relief of sneezing, itching and rhinorrhea, but as discussed earlier, they are less effective than inhaled topical glucocorticoid sprays in controlling symptoms of rhinitis. When using antihistamines, second generation formulations are preferred as they have less sedative and anticholinergic properties. Nasal antihistamine sprays, azelastine and olopatadine, are used in the management of AR as they have an anti-inflammatory effect and are equally efficacious in relieving symptoms of nasal obstruction.[11-13] Topical antihistamines are a useful adjunct to oral glucocorticoids, and comparable to oral antihistamines with their onset of action occurring within 15 minutes.[14] Cromolyn sodium is a mast cell stabilizer by inhibiting chloride channels on the cell surface and prevents the release of histamine and other mediators of allergic inflammation. It is more effective than placebo in alleviating AR symptoms with minimal side effects, but is not as effective as antihistamines and topic glucocorticoids.[5,15,16] Cromolyn should be administered 30 minutes prior to allergen exposure as it alleviates symptoms during the immediate phases of an allergic reaction. It is useful in patients who only have intermittent exposures to allergens.

Topical decongestants are not recommended in the treatment of AR as they are prone to tachyphylaxis by down-regulating the alpha-adrenergic receptor, leading to worsening rebound congestion (rhinitis medicamentosa). Combination of an oral antihistamine and decongestant is more effective than oral antihistamines, but is limited in its use due to adverse side effects of the oral decongestant. Their availability is now limited in the United States due to the use of pseudoephedrine as a stimulant and in the production of methamphetamine. In over-the-counter products, pseudoephedrine has been replaced by phenylephrine, which is not as efficacious in relieving the symptoms of rhinitis, and may not even be better than placebo. Short course of oral glucocorticoids, shown to be more effective than placebo,[17,18] may be used as a last resort in AR when other treatments are insufficient or symptoms are severe enough to impair sleep and the ability to work.[14,19]

## Nonallergic Rhinitis

The distinguishing presentation of nonallergic rhinitis from allergic is generally the absence of sneezing and allergic conjunctivitis, particularly the lack of red, itchy and watery eyes.

*Occupational rhinitis*: Exposure to environmental toxins such as chemicals or smoke causes direct damage to the nasal mucosa resulting in occupational rhinitis (OR). Typical irritants include dust, ozone, sulfur dioxide, ammonia and cigarette smoke, which produce nasal congestion, dryness, rhinorrhea, nasal pruritus and sneezing. Healthcare workers, cleaners, bakers, apprentices in high-risk occupations, and workers exposed to multiple agents are at highest risk of OR.[20] Environmental controls and limiting further exposure are the only treatment options.

*Hormonal rhinitis*: Hormonal mediated rhinitis (HR) affects women in pregnancy and its incidence is greater than 20%. HR due to increased circulating estrogens causing increased tissue swelling and congestion by increased nasal hyaluronic acid deposition and vascular engorgement. Furthermore, estrogen and progesterone increases expression of H1 receptors and eosinophil migration and degranulation. In addition, there is an enlargement of mucous glands and decreased cilia, which limits mucus clearance, contributing to congestion usually during the second and third trimesters.[21,22]

*Drug-induced rhinitis*: Drug-induced rhinitis is mediated by local inflammation, neurogenic, or sometimes even unknown mechanisms. Typically implicated medications include beta-blockers, alpha-blockers, angiotensin converting enzyme (ACE) inhibitors, calcium channel blockers, thiazide diuretics, methyldopa, hydralazine, phosphodiesterase inhibitors, tricyclic antidepressants, and benzodiazepines. Treatment is generally discontinuing or substituting the offending medications. Symptomatic treatment initially with intranasal corticosteroids and adding intranasal antihistamine, if initial treatment is ineffective, is a reasonable approach.[23] *Rhinitis medicamentosa*: Alpha-adrenergic agonists, found in topical vasoconstrictors such as oxymetazoline, cause decongestion by activating alpha-2 receptors. However, use longer than 3–5 days leads to down-regulation of the alpha-adrenergic receptors and produces rebound congestion. This leads to a cycle of nasal congestion that is both caused by and temporarily relieved by the medication. The result is often an escalating use of decongestants.

*Nonallergic rhinitis with eosinophilia syndrome (NARES)*: NARES presents with symptoms consistent with AR, watery rhinorrhea, and nasal pruritus without atopy. Anosmia is a distinguishing feature from AR. NARES affects 15% of patients with nonallergic rhinitis and is usually associated with more severe exacerbations predisposing to sinusitis, polyposis, sleep apnea, and aspirin sensitivity. Eosinophilia greater than 20% on nasal smear with negative allergen testing, either skin or serum IgE assays characterizes this syndrome. Treatment is usually symptomatic with intranasal corticosteroids with or without antihistamines.[24]

## Rhinosinusitis

Rhinosinusitis is the inflammation of the nasal mucosa and paranasal sinuses and is largely used interchangeably with sinusitis.[25] In acute rhinosinusitis, the episode lasts less than 4 weeks, and is defined as chronic if symptoms persist for more than 12 weeks. Symptomatic episodes lasting 4–12 weeks are defined as sub-acute. Rhinosinusitis is quite common and it affects one in six adults in the United States.[1] Most cases of acute rhinosinusitis are due to viral infections and generally resolve in 7–10 days, but bacterial superinfection complicates up to 2% of cases. Chronic rhinosinusitis is thought to result from mucosal inflammation leading to swelling and obstruction of the sinuses leading to mucus stasis, which may result in superinfection. There are a variety of causes of chronic rhinosinusitis, such as osteitis, allergies, infectious superantigens and biofilms, and host immunodeficiency. Bony inflammation in chronic sinusitis is known to occur and the bones of the paranasal sinuses can undergo remodeling secondary to chronic inflammation despite aggressive mucosal anti-inflammatory treatment. Some believe the chronic, persistent inflammation in the bones seen in osteitis, maybe the etiology of some cases of intractable chronic rhinosinusitis. Further, allergy is more prevalent among patients with chronic rhinosinusitis, and may contribute to the pathophysiology, though the mechanism remains unknown. More recently, research has shown the existence of biofilms from pathogens such as *Pseudomonas aeruginosa*, *Staphylococcus aureus*, and *Haemophilus influenzae* may play a causative role in refractory chronic rhinosinusitis. Some research has also shown that superantigens released by *S. aureus*, may lead to immune system activation and subsequent inflammation contributing top chronic rhinosinusitis and polyp formation.[26] Moreover, fungal hyphae have been fond in the 96% of patients with chronic rhinosinusitis, which may up regulate interleukin (IL)-5 and IL-13 causing eosinophil recruitment and proliferation resulting in chronic rhinosinusitis.[27,28] Lastly, immune deficiency can predispose patients to diffuse inflammation leading to chronic rhinosinusitis, studies have shown that more than 60% of patients with human immunodeficiency virus (HIV) will suffer from some degree of rhinosinusitis.

*Presentation*: Rhinosinusitis typically presents with nasal obstruction, mucopurulent discharge, and facial fullness or sinus tenderness. Other symptoms that may be present include fever, fatigue, anosmia, halitosis, ear pressure and headache. Distinguishing between bacterial and viral causes on clinical criteria alone is often difficult. Generally, in viral rhinosinusitis, symptoms last less than 7–10 days and whose progression is typically stable, whereas in bacterial rhinosinusitis, symptoms persist more than 7–10 days and worsen after initial period of improvement—indicating a secondary infectious insult. Red flag signs and symptoms for urgent referral and imaging include high-grade fevers (>39°C), severe headache, vision abnormalities, and peri-orbital edema, as they may indicate intracranial and/or orbital extension.

*Diagnosis*: Have the patient bend forward to elicit focal sinus pain, percuss sinuses to elicit pain, and examine the oropharynx for a red streak to aide in confirming the diagnosis.[29] On anterior rhinoscopy mucosal edema and purulence can aide the diagnosis and anatomic deformities such as inferior turbinate hypertrophy (ITH), narrowing of the middle meatus, deviated septum or polyps may predispose or complicate rhinosinusitis. Diagnostic imaging in the initial evaluation of rhinosinusitis is unnecessary except when red flag symptoms are present, in resistant or recurrent cases (>3–4 episodes annually), or when considering other suspicious etiologies.[30] Sinus radiography is 87% sensitive and 89% specific in diagnosing sinusitis, but viral and bacterial sinusitis appears similarly on radiographs.[31] Computed tomography (CT) is the imaging modality of choice over sinus radiography to visualize the sinuses. It is superior in its ability to visualize bony and soft tissue structures facilitating the assessment for air-fluid levels. When there is concern for resistant bacterial species or guidance for antibiotic management is needed, endoscopic examination to obtain accurate middle meatus cultures by an otolaryngologist is warranted to improve diagnostic yield as they have good sensitivity (81%) and specificity (91%), with a high positive predictive value (83%).[32] Nasal swab cultures have no role in diagnosis as they do not reflect the pathogens in the sinuses.

*Treatment*: The goals of treatment for acute rhinosinusitis vary according to its infectious etiology and 40–60% of cases of acute bacterial rhinosinusitis will resolve without intervention. The objective of treatment in acute viral rhinosinusitis is to relieve symptoms, while in acute bacterial rhinosinusitis it is to resolve the infection and prevent complications. Either watchful waiting or antibiotic treatment in mild acute bacterial rhinosinusitis at day 10 of symptoms is reasonable. Treatment with antibiotics should be initiated for moderate-severe symptomatic cases of bacterial rhinosinusitis. The antibiotic of choice in most patients is amoxicillin with optimal duration varying from short courses (3–6 days) to long courses (7–10 days), although some studies have shown little difference between the short and long courses.[33] For adults a 5–7 day course is recommended, while a longer course is recommended for children.[34] Furthermore, concern for resistant *Moraxella catarrhalis* or *H. influenzae* requires the addition of clavulanic acid or a different class of antibiotics. Trimethoprim-sulfamethoxazole, macrolides, and second- and third-generation oral cephalosporins are reasonable alternative first-line agents in patients with penicillin allergies.[35-37]

Treatment failure is defined as worsening of symptoms at anytime after initiating therapy, or by lack of improvement in symptoms within 7 days. When treatment failure occurs, a broader spectrum antibiotic should be used and consideration should be made to refer to and otolaryngologist in order to obtain cultures. Symptomatic treatment is indicated for both acute bacterial and viral rhinosinusitis, which consists of analgesics, saline irrigations, topical steroids, antihistamines, mucolytics, topical, and oral decongestants. Nonsteroidal anti-inflammatory drugs (NSAIDs) and acetaminophen are recommended for pain control. Mechanical nasal irrigation with sterile buffered isotonic saline may improve patient comfort by providing symptom relief and decrease the need for pain medications.[38] Topical steroids for 2–3 weeks have minimal adverse reactions and decrease mucosal inflammation, and successfully relieve symptoms of sinonasal obstruction.[39] Antihistamines have a role in the treatment of atopic patients with acute rhinosinusitis, as they improve symptoms such as sneezing and nasal obstruction, but have not been shown to be of benefit in nonatopic patients and can have side effects including drowsiness, headache and xerostomia.[40,41] Decongestants decrease nasal congestion, particularly at the inferior and middle turbinates, improve mucosal inflammation, subjectively improve nasal obstruction, and improve mucociliary clearance.[42-45] Decongestants should be used sparingly and for no more than 3 consecutive days to avoid rebound congestion.[46] Topical decongestants may be useful, but have never been proven to be more effective than simple saline irrigation.[47,48] Mucolytics such as guaifenesin can assist in drainage of mucous by thinning secretions, but their use in rhinosinusitis has not been FDA approved or studied.[47]

## Chronic Rhinosinusitis

There is lack of quality data for the management of chronic rhinosinusitis secondary to the heterogeneity of recommendations, however, a combined treatment with a short taper of oral corticosteroids for 10–15 days and 3–4 weeks of antibiotics with adjunctive saline irrigation and topical corticosteroids is appropriate.[49-51] Antibiotic course may be extended to 6 weeks if the improvement is gradual and there is not an indication for surgery. Maintenance therapy usually consists of topical corticosteroid and saline irrigation until symptomatic improvement.[52] Surgical management via functional endoscopic sinus surgery (FESS) can be the next step in management following the failure of medical treatment as it works to restore sinus ventilation by ensuring ostial patency. FESS is also indicated for the removal of material from opacified sinuses, debulking of severe polyposis, removal of inspissated mucin in allergic fungal rhinosinusitis, bony erosion, and extension of disease beyond the sinus cavity. In cases where surgery is performed, it is important to continue medical therapy concomitantly, as surgery does not address the underlying inflammatory condition.

## Anatomic Variation

Normal airflow begins in the nostrils as negative air pressure brings air through the nasal passage to the choanae, passing through the turbinates, septum, and ostiomeatal complex. This process causes the typical turbulence that is perceived as the normal sensation of airflow. Anatomic variations can lead to altered flow or perception of altered flow resulting in the symptoms of nasal obstruction.

## Septal Perforation or Other Intranasal Structural Loss

Septal perforations can present with symptoms of nasal obstruction, crusting, discharge, epistaxis, and whistling on nasal breathing. A thorough history should be performed to elicit a potential history of trauma, recent medications, any infectious process, presence of any systemic diseases, or exposure to toxic substances. External trauma to the nasal septum can result in a hematoma formation, which can lead to ischemia and eventually necrosis. Digital manipulation can result in self-inflicted trauma and septal perforation. In addition iatrogenic trauma from septoplasty, nasal packing, cauterization, nasal intubation, or nasogastric tube placement can perforate the septum. Medication use should be reviewed, as nasal decongestants and even intranasal glucocorticoid sprays have been reported to cause septal perforations. Furthermore, the use of illicit intranasal drugs, such as cocaine and pain medications, should be elicited.[53] Tuberculosis, syphilis, HIV, and fungal infections, as well as systemic disease like sarcoidosis, granulomatosis with polyangiitis, systemic lupus erythematosus, rheumatoid arthritis, or other collagen vascular diseases, may cause a perforated septum.[54,55] Exposure to toxic industrial fumes, wood dust, leather tanning and nickel refining process increases the risk of developing septal perforation. On external examination of the nose, assess for saddle nose deformity as perforation may result in loss of cartilaginous support. On anterior rhinoscopy, crusting may be present and should be removed to fully visualize the nasal septum. Th entire septum should be visualized and will likely require endoscopy (Fig. 1). Posterior perforations are more likely to be asymptomatic in comparison to anterior perforations. Referral to otolaryngologist for nasal biopsy of the perforated edge should be performed to rule out a neoplastic etiology. When a septal perforation is present, it is important to keep the nose moist to prevent crusting. Petroleum jelly, nasal emollients, nasal irrigation, or a humidifier can be helpful. Surgery can be performed to relieve symptoms. In symptomatic patients who prefer to avoid surgery, a prosthetic can be inserted in the office with local anesthesia to occlude the perforation.

## Septal Deviation

Septal deviation is one of the most common causes of nasal obstruction, as it is easily damaged with even minor blunt trauma. Risk factors for it include traumatic or forceps delivery in infants, and accidental trauma in adults. Chronic unilateral congestion increases the suspicion for deviated septum, particularly with a history of trauma, even if remote or minor. Anterior nasal septal deviations

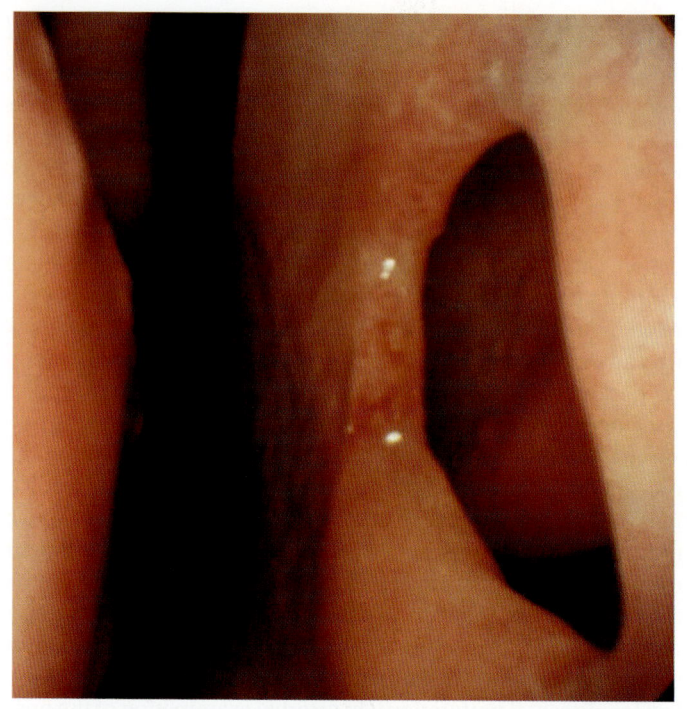

**Fig. 1:** Endoscopic view of septal perforation.

are known to be more problematic to the patient and cause greater symptoms than posterior nasal septal deviations (Fig. 2). Visualization of a laterally deviated septum on anterior rhinoscopy or palpation of a deviated septum on examination of the external nose establishes the diagnosis. However, if the history is convincing and anterior rhinoscopy or physical examination does not establish the diagnosis, it is appropriate to refer patients to an otolaryngologist for an endoscopic nasal examination. Treatment is typically geared at alleviating the deviated septum via a surgical procedure called a septoplasty. It is critical to counsel patients about when and to what degree of symptomatic improvement they may expect following the procedure. Studies have reported variable long-term efficacy, but in general, significant improvement is usually seen by 6 months, and up to 90% of patients report improvement in their obstructive symptoms.[56]

## Inferior Turbinate Hypertrophy

Inferior turbinate hypertrophy causes increased resistance due to both its anatomic position and size. ITH also occurs secondary

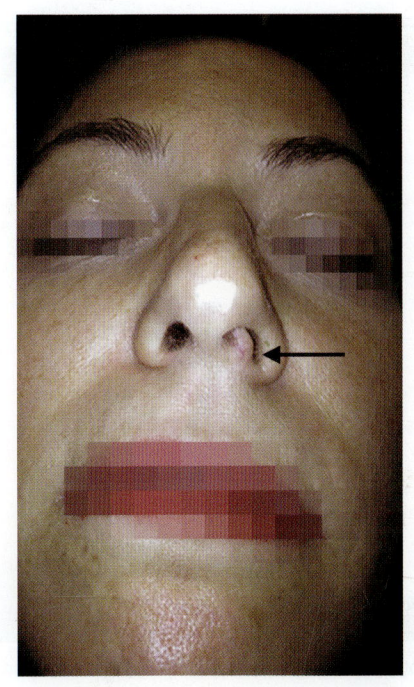

**Fig. 2:** This is a demonstration of septal deviation. Arrow marks the prominent caudal septum.

to soft tissue or mucosal inflammation in allergic rhinitis, nonallergic rhinitis, and rhinitis medicamentosa making it potentially responsive to medical therapy. However, following chronic mucosal inflammation, mucous glands can hypertrophy, leading to irreversible enlargement. In addition, bony hypertrophy may also occur resulting in ITH as well, often due to septal deviation. Septal deviation causes alteration of resistance and airflow in one nasal cavity and thus the inferior nasal turbinate hypertrophies in order to compensate for the decreased airflow. Diagnose ITH by using anterior rhinoscopy, or endoscopically (Fig. 3) to visualize enlarged inferior turbinates. Initial treatment generally utilizes antihistamines, intranasal steroids, and topical decongestants to decrease mucosal and soft tissue inflammation to relieve the nasal obstruction. If medical management is unsuccessful, surgical options include inferior turbinate reduction.

## Nasal Valve Collapse

Resistance to airflow caused by the nose is quite significant, and can account for up to 50% of the resistance that needs to be overcome

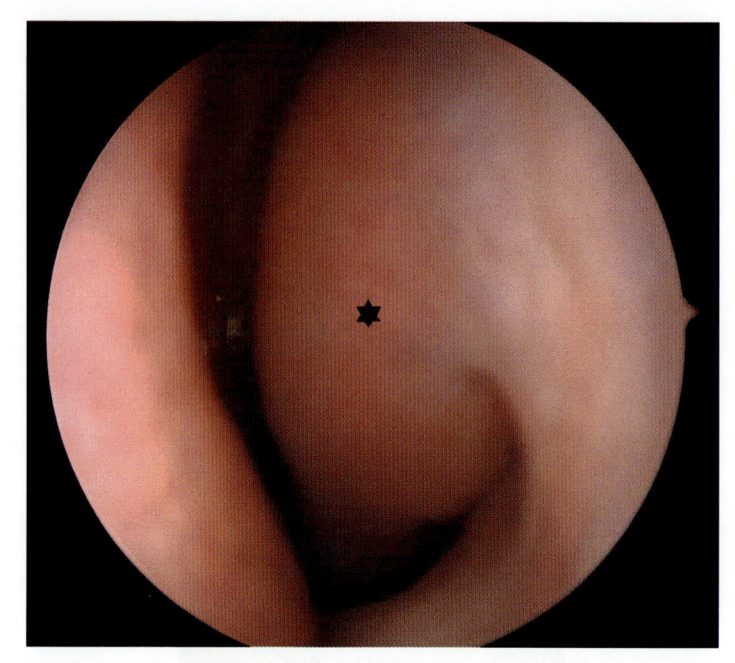

**Fig. 3:** Endoscopic view of inferior turbinate hypertrophy. The asterisk marks the inferior turbinate.

on inspiration.[57] The nasal valve is the narrowest part of the nasal airway, thus based on Poiseuille's law that airflow through a tube is inversely proportional to the radius to the fourth power this is an area of high airflow. Subsequently based on Bernoulli's principle that as airflow increases, the intraluminal pressure decreases, this is the region of lowest intraluminal pressure. Therefore, it follows that small deviations in the anatomy can result in dramatic changes in airflow and intraluminal pressure. So it follows that airflow is rapid through a narrow area, such as the nasal valve, the intraluminal pressure decreases and allows valve collapse and dysfunction if the structural integrity is weakened for any reason.

There are two types of nasal valve dysfunction resulting from different etiologies. The first is dysfunction in the area surrounding the valve, while the second is due to nasal valve collapse, a common complication of rhinoplasty and aging, as both weaken the nasal sidewalls. The most common etiology of nasal valve dysfunction is rhinoplasty, as overly aggressive osteotomies leads to medial displacement of the nasal bones and its attached upper lateral cartilage, collapsing the valve. Furthermore, over-resection of the lower lateral cartilage can weaken the area and cause collapse on inspiration.

Other causes of collapse include Mohs excision of dermatologic malignancies damaging the cartilage and facial paralysis. Nasal valve collapse is diagnosed by seeing a pinched tip or hourglass figure at the middle segment of the nose. Collapse of the ala following deep inspiration also is diagnostic of nasal valve collapse. Furthermore, the Cottle's maneuver evaluates nasal valve patency. In this maneuver, two fingers pull laterally against the cheek and the evaluator assesses for improvement in nasal breathing and patency. Performing anterior rhinoscopy after the application of topical decongestant allows the practitioner to visualize if nasal obstruction can be relieved. Ifdecongestants relieve obstruction, aggressive medical therapy may alleviate the need for surgical correction. Surgical correction of nasal valve collapse with reconstructive surgery generally requires the placements of small grafts to buttress the valve, or flaring/ suspension sutures to open the valve.[58]

## Bilateral or Unilateral Choanal Atresia

Choanal atresia is a congenital obstruction of the posterior orifice of the nasal cavity that can result from both bony as well as mixed bony-membranous atresia. It may occur bilaterally and present in infancy with respiratory distress and cyclical cyanosis that improves with crying and deteriorates with feeding, as neonates are obligate nasal breathers. Unilateral choanal atresia (Fig. 4) occurs more commonly on the right and may present later in life with obstruction. CT scan is the imaging modality of choice to characterize the anatomic deformity, but is often discovered when a practitioner is unable to pass a catheter or endoscope. Initial treatment, especially of bilateral choanal atresia requires securing a safe airway with either an oral airway, McGovern nipple, or intubation until surgical correction of the atresia can occur by a specialist.

## Nasal Pyriform Aperture Stenosis

Congenital nasal pyriform aperture stenosis may present similarly to choanal atresia depending on its severity and is characterized by bony overgrowth of the medial maxilla, narrowing the nasal inlet. In severe cases, it appears similar to bilateral choanal atresia with respiratory distress and cyclical cyanosis that improves with crying and deteriorates with feeding. Establishing a secure and safe airway is critical, and if mild, symptomatic treatment with suctioning, topical decongestants, and intranasal corticosteroids may be tried, with resolution as the child grows. However, surgical repair is warranted if medical therapy fails, the child loses weight, or has respiratory distress.

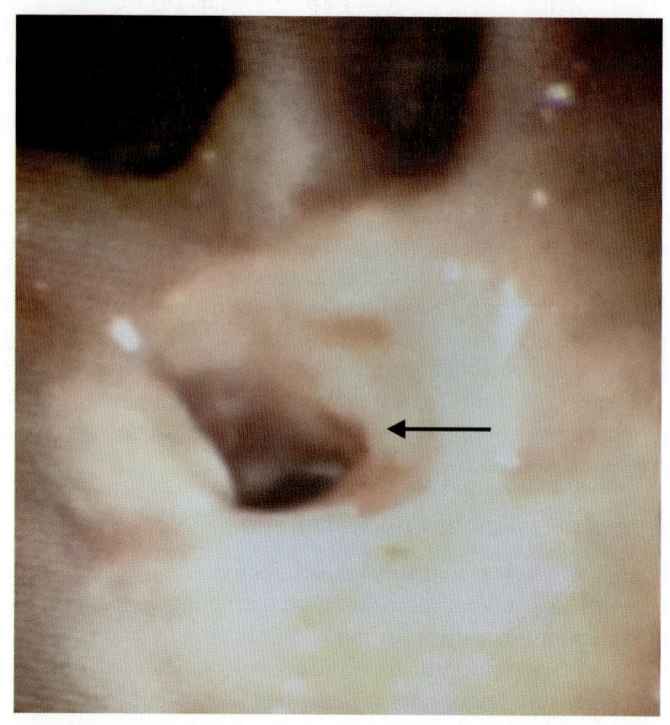

**Fig. 4:** Endoscopic view, choanal atresia. The arrow marks the stenosis or narrowing of the choanae after repair of the choanal atresia.

## Concha Bullosa

Concha bullosa is pneumatization of the turbinates, that usually occurs in the medial or superior turbinates. The incidence ranges from 14% to 53% on endoscopic examination.[59] It is one of the most common variants of sinonasal anatomy. In some studies, prevalence of concha bullosa is up to 80% in chronic sinusitis and has been shown to be more prevalent in these cases rather than controls, indicating it may play a role in its pathogenesis, due to its size.[60-62] Treatment is generally FESS with a goal of remitting symptoms.

## Nasal Masses

Patients who present with sinonasal masses typically present with nasal obstruction and thus make up an important segment of patients presenting with nasal obstruction. Other presenting symptoms include rhinorrhea, hyposmia, epistaxis and headache. The majority of masses are nonneoplastic, but up to 40% have the potential to be neoplastic. About half will present with unilateral mass and complaints, while the remaining half will have bilateral masses.[63,64]

## Congenital Midline Nasal Masses

Congenital midline nasal masses are uncommon lesions that occur at the nasal bridge and extend intranasal and intracranial to communicate with the subarachnoid space. The more common lesions are nasal dermoids, nasal glial heterotopias and encephaloceles. All congenital midline nasal masses warranting a thorough evaluation must exclude other congenital anomalies. Manipulation of the mass should be avoided. Neuroimaging is required to determine specific type of lesion, delineate the presence and extent of intracranial extension, and allow surgical planning.[65,66] Magnetic resonance imaging (MRI) is generally preferred to evaluate intracranial involvement, but CT may be helpful in determining osseous defects that would affect the surgical plan.[67] If intracranial extension is suspected clinically or on radiography, neurosurgical consultation is warranted for intracranial resection and otolaryngology consultation for external resection.[68]

*Dacrocystoceles* or nasolacrimal duct cysts occur when the nasolacrimal duct fails to canalize during embryonic development. The obstruction of tear drainage leads to dilation of the nasolacrimal duct. It usually presents with unilateral epiphora especially during the first year of life.[69] A defect in the nasolacrimal duct occurs in 5–6% of newborns.[70] Patients may also present with nasal pathology such as an intranasal cyst, which can cause nasal obstruction and even respiratory distress. Imaging with CT scan is the modality of choice to visualize a cystic mass at the medial canthus or at the inferior turbinate. Treatment with topical decongestants for mild symptoms such as epiphora is reasonable. Severe symptoms and nasal obstruction are treated with endoscopic resection or dacryocystorhinostomy tube placement.[71]

## Benign Neoplasms

Many different benign lesions may occur in the nasal cavity and despite their inability to metastasize they can cause significant local destruction and have high rates of local recurrence. Visualization on endoscopy and early referral to otolaryngology for surgical management leads to reduced morbidity and faster recovery.[72]

*Inverted papilloma*: Inverted papilloma (IP), also called a schneiderian papilloma, is benign lesion of the nasal cavity that is locally aggressive and has a tendency for recurrence if not adequately excised. There is an association with malignancy, particularly squamous cell carcinoma (SCC) likely through alterations in p53 and or HPV infection.[73] IPs characteristically originate from the lateral nasal wall close to the middle meatus in over 90% of cases and have a granular berry type appearance, but can also occur in the septum. Only a small portion of the lesion is visible, as it tends to invert into the surrounding tissue and can involve the paranasal sinuses. Treatment with endoscopic surgical resection is feasible in about two-thirds of cases, and when not feasible open surgical resection is the treatment of choice.[74]

*Fibro-osseous lesions and osteomas*: Ossifying fibromas are benign tumors that are usually incidentally found on radiographic imaging during 2nd to 4th decades of life and have a strong female predilection. Ossifying fibromas have a predilection for the mandible, but may also be found in the paranasal sinuses. Osteomas, however, are the most common benign tumor of the paranasal sinuses usually presenting in the 2nd to 3rd decade of life, more commonly affecting men. Fibro-osseous lesions replace normal bone with tissues comprised of fibroblasts and collagen with a variable amount of mineralization and is thought that trauma and inflammation play a role in their formation. Ossifying fibromas are usually slow growing and rarely cause symptoms by mass effect or nasal obstruction, but may become unpredictably aggressive, especially when located paranasally. These lesions may be identified on endoscopic examination and surgically resected if they become symptomatic.

*Angiofibromas*: Juvenile nasopharyngeal angiofibromas (JNAs) (Fig. 5) are benign locally invasive vascular neoplasms that tend to grow slowly. They predominantly occur in adolescent males in the nasal cavity extending into the nasopharynx, but have been reported in other locations as well.[75] JNAs typically present with recurrent epistaxis and unilateral nasal congestion. They typically form at the sphenopalatine foramen and can proceed to have extradural intracranial extension. JNAs may regress spontaneously in certain cases and are rare in adults, thus surgical management should be reserved for significant symptoms such as recurrent nosebleeds and persistent nasal obstruction. On endoscopic examination, they appear as a pale-pink to beefy red lobulated mass in the nasopharynx or nasal cavity. Imaging with CT, MRI, or magnetic resonance angiography (MRA) is helpful in delineating intracranial involvement.

*Pyogenic granuloma*: Pyogenic granulomas (PGs) are benign vascular neoplasms that ironically are not pyogenic nor granulomatous

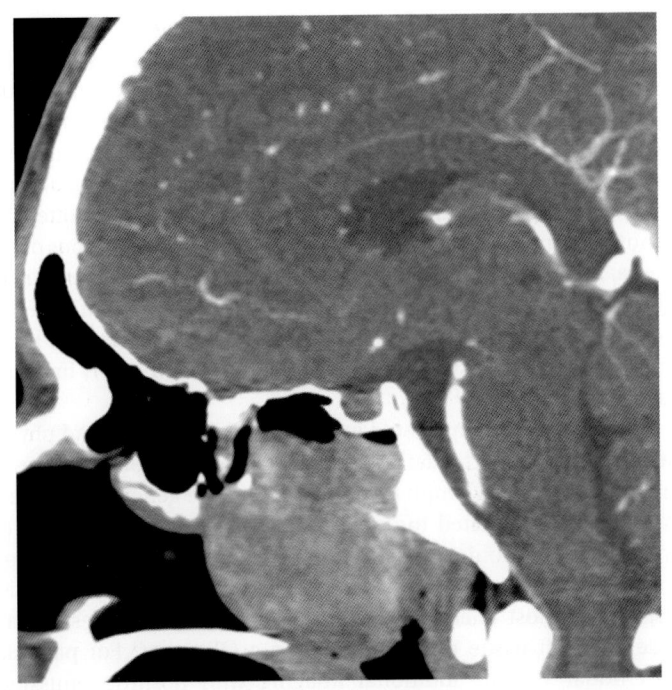

**Fig. 5:** Sagittal CT scan of benign sinonasal tumor, juvenile nasopharyngeal angiofibroma.

on histology. PGs predominantly occur on the gingiva, but can also present in the nasal cavity as well. They usually present with a rapidly growing, red to purple hued solitary mass, recurrent epistaxis, and nasal obstruction similar to JNAs.[76] PGs are responsive to hormone stimulation and often appear during pregnancy, usually during the second and third trimesters, at the site of former trauma and regress to a fibroma following parturition.[77] Treatment generally consists of a combination of excision with electrodessication, silver nitrate, cryotherapy, and pulsed dye or argon lasers maybe used as well. Indications for surgical resection are usually severe symptoms, recurrent bleeding, or failure to resolve with parturition.[78] Recurrence frequently occurs with incomplete resection.[79]

## Nasopharyngeal Cancer

In the United States, the annual incidence of nasopharyngeal carcinomas is less than 2 per 100,000 with a two- to three-fold higher incidence in males with a peak incidence during 5th and 6th decades of life. The incidence is much higher in Southeast Asia, Middle East, and North Africa and is endemic in Southern China. Persons from these regions retain the higher risk profile even when they migrate into low risk areas. The etiology is multifactorial, with environmental and genetic influences including HLA (human leukocyte antigen)-BW46, HLA-B17, ingestion of preserved foods that release nitrosamine like salted or cured fish, and exposure to Epstein-Barr virus (EBV).[80-82] The earliest symptoms of nasopharyngeal cancers such as epistaxis, rhinorrhea or nasal obstruction can often go unnoticed, and can present with a neck mass, refractory serous otitis media, and headache due to cranial nerve (CN) involvement, usually CN III–VI. Unfortunately, since a substantial portion of patients will remain asymptomatic initially, a significant majority will have lymph node metastasis at the time of diagnosis and nearly half will have bilateral spread.

Diagnostic work up should include a detailed history and physical examination, particularly a thorough CN evaluation and assessment of the cervical lymph nodes. EBV titers are generally elevated in poorly differentiated tumors and maybe used for establishing prognosis and noninvasive monitoring for recurrence.[83] Endoscopic visualization and biopsy can definitively establish the diagnosis. MRI is the most effective imaging modality for these lesions as it defines soft tissue much superior to a CT scan.[84] For patients with nodal spread, additional imaging with positron emission tomography (PET) scan is recommended to assess for metastasis.[85] In cases where a PET scan is not feasible, a bone scan or CT imaging of the CT and abdomen should be considered. Given the difficulty of obtaining clean margins surgically, the primary treatment is generally radiation therapy, which includes bilateral neck and supraclavicular lymph nodes.

## Sinonasal Tumors

Given the anatomic proximity of the nasal cavity to the paranasal sinuses, it is often difficult to define the origin of these masses. Since they have similar histopathology and treatments, they are generally grouped together. Sinonasal tumors are more prevalent in men and tend to present in the 5th to 6th decades of life. Exposures to tobacco smoke, wood dust, and leather tanning have been associated with the development of nasal cavity tumors. These tumors tend to present with unilateral nasal obstruction, nasal discharge, epistaxis, and facial pain mimicking the signs and symptoms of chronic rhinosinusitis. Sinonasal tumors are locally damaging, but lymph node metastasis occurs in less than 10%. Obtaining tissue biopsy by nasal endoscopy can establish the definitive pathologic diagnosis. SCC is the most common pathologic finding, but minor salivary gland adenocarcinomas, neuroendocrine carcinomas, melanomas, lymphomas, and sarcomas are other possible etiologies. Imaging with both CT and MRI is performed, as CT is better able to evaluate the bony structures in detail, while MRI better visualizes invasion into the soft tissues, orbit and cranium. Treatment usually involves a multidisciplinary approach with surgical resection and pre- and post-operative radiation therapy. Follow-up intensity is the greatest for the first 4 years as the vast majority of local recurrences will occur during this period. CT with contrast imaging is the modality of choice when monitoring for recurrence as it visualizes lymph nodes superior than MRI.

*Squamous cell carcinoma*: SCC are the most common type of sinonasal tumor and most likely to arise from the lateral nasal wall. They account for nearly 50% of the tumors found in the nasal cavity.[86] The prognosis of these tumors is related to the extent of their spread and location. Early TNM stage tumors are generally treated with surgical excision or radiation therapy; however, advanced stage tumors are treated with a multidisciplinary approach, most commonly surgical excision followed by radiation or chemoradiation therapy. The 5-year overall survival rate is only around 50–60%.[87,88]

*Adenocarcinoma*: Adenocarcinomas account for less than 10% of all sinonasal tumors and have a strong male predominance, 80–90%. They are epidemiologically associated with hardwood dust exposure. The histologic grade and tumor growth pattern affect prognosis. Papillary lesions are localized and have a good prognosis, whereas sessile lesions are invasive, and alveolal mucoid lesions are the most aggressive. Low-grade lesions are highly differentiated and rarely have distant metastasis, but tend to recur locally with a 75% 5-year survival. High-grade lesions have high mitotic activity and metastatic disease is often present at the time of diagnosis with over 60% of patients dying within three years.[89] Treatment is generally surgical resection with the addition of radiation therapy for advanced lesions or those resected without clean margins.[90]

*Minor salivary gland tumors*: Adenoid cystic carcinomas (ACC) are the most common type of minor salivary gland tumors, which are most commonly found in the maxillary sinuses followed by the nasal cavity. ACCs rarely metastasize regionally via lymphatic spread, but commonly invade neurovascular structures and may spread intracranially and hematogenously. The 5-year overall survival rate with ACC is approximately 60%, however long-term follow-up is critical as late recurrence is common. Treatment is generally surgical excision with the addition of radiation therapy for involved surgical margins or advanced and high-grade tumors.[91]

*Ethesioneuroblastoma*: Ethesioneuroblastomas (ENBs) are olfactory neuroblastomas (Fig. 6) which arise from the olfactory epithelium in the superior nasal vault which account for up to 5–13% of nasal cavity tumors.[86] They have a bimodal distribution of incidence, with peak incidence at 10–20 years of age and then again during the 6th decades of life. ENB prognosis relates to the extent of disease present on diagnosis and the ability to perform surgical resection. Treatment is usually with endoscopic surgical resection followed by radiation therapy.[92]

*Mucosal melanoma*: Melanomas are generally rapidly lethal neoplasms and though less than 1% of all melanomas arise from the sinonasal tract.[86] Melanomas of the sinonasal tract are found in the nasal cavity most commonly at the nasal septum and inferior turbinates. Prognosis is related to the thickness of the lesion. Most melanomas are at an advanced stage due to the depth of invasion. In addition, nearly a third will have neck metastases, which is generally considered a marker of distant spread. Local recurrence is common as more than half of patients will have local recurrence and likely

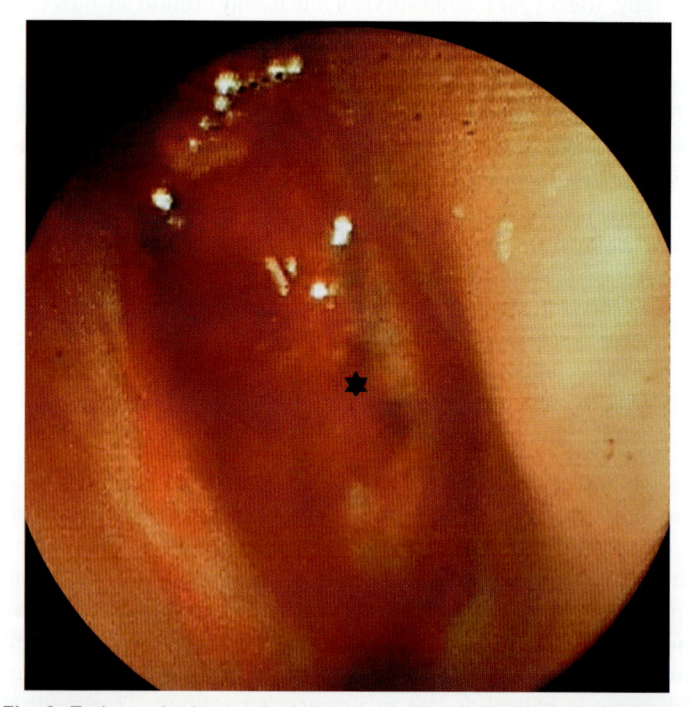

**Fig. 6:** Endoscopic view, malignant tumor, esthesioneuroblastoma. Note the bleeding and ulceration present. The asterisk marks the tumor-esthesioneuroblastoma.

distant metastases soon after, which can be rapidly fatal.[93] Treatment is surgical resection with the possible addition of radiation therapy to assist in gaining local control, though radiation therapy does not seem to affect overall survival.[93,94]

## Infectious Etiologies

*Rhinoscleroma* is the result of granulomatous inflammation of the upper respiratory tract caused by an infection from a *Klebsiella pneumoniae.* subspecies rhinoscleromatis or ozaenae. It is rare in Europe and the United States, but is endemic in North and Central Africa, Southeast Asia, and South and Central America.[95,96] It is thought that poor hygiene and nutritional deficiencies contribute to the acquisition of this disease.[97] Rhinoscleroma tends to occur in younger patients, generally aged 10–30. Patients with rhinoscleroma have impaired cellular immunity as evidenced by decreased levels of CD4 cells and altered CD4/CD8 ratio in the lesion. Nasal rhinoscleroma occurs in three typical stages, catarrhal, proliferative, and cicatricial stages. Rhinoscleroma typically presents with symptoms similar to rhinitis in the catarrhal stage and is often misdiagnosed. Nasal obstruction and rhinorrhea are the most common complaint, but mucopurulent discharge, epistaxis, crusting, scarring leading to occlusion of the nasolacrimal duct, and bony and cartilaginous deformity caused by granulomatous nodules occur in later stages of the disease.[98]

Nasal endoscopy is recommended to visualize the lesions and obtaining samples to isolate the bacterium by culture. Serology has also been used to obtain a diagnosis. CT imaging is the radiographic modality of choice to examine the extent of lesion. Rhinoscleroma is generally sensitive to most common antibiotics with ciprofloxacin and rifampin having the most activity against the bacteria.[98] Given the high rates of recurrence, close follow-up and long-term antibiotics are often needed. Surgery may be considered alongside antibiotics in the cases when granulomatous nodules and significant symptoms of obstruction are present.

*Rhinosporidiosis*: Rhinosporidiosis is chronic granulomatous infection caused by a water parasite, *Rhinosporidium seeberi*. It presents as a vascular, friable polyp arising from the nasal mucosa causing symptoms of unilateral nasal obstruction, epistaxis, coryza, rhinorrhea, postnasal drip, or a foreign body sensation.[99,100] It is endemic in India and Sri Lanka, and occurs predominantly in young men, but in the United States it is seen, albeit rarely, in Texas and the

Southeast. Visualizing the organism's typical features on microscopy with fungal stains or potassium hydroxide establishes the diagnosis, as these organisms are difficult to grow in vitro. CT imaging may be helpful in determining the site and extent of disease.[101] Rhinosporidiosis is treated with surgical excision, as these lesions do not respond well to medical treatment, although dapsone has been successful in some cases.[102]

## Autoimmune Etiologies

A chronic systemic inflammatory state generally characterizes granulomatous and autoimmune diseases and many of these disorders have sinonasal manifestations. These autoimmune diseases include granulomatosis with polyangiitis, sarcoidosis, Churg-Strauss, and T-Cell lymphoma. Early appearances of systemic disease are generally nonspecific and include nasal obstruction, rhinorrhea, and recurrent episodes of rhinosinusitis. A brief description of these diseases and their role in symptomatic nasal obstruction can be found in Table 1.

# Polyposis

Sinonasal polyps (Fig. 7) are one of the most common nasal masses and affect nearly 4% of the population. The etiology remains unknown, however polyps are associated with allergies, asthma, aspirin sensitivity, cystic fibrosis, primary ciliary dyskinesia, and infections.[103] Polyposis is a multifactorial disease in which chronic inflammation plays a significant role. Chronic inflammatory states lead to mucosal inflammation and edema which can cause prolapse into the nasal cavity causing symptoms of nasal obstruction, rhinorrhea, post nasal drip, anosmia, and sometimes headache.[104] A thorough history should be obtained, especially seeking out potential allergic etiologies. On anterior rhinoscopy, polyps may be visualized, but endoscopy with decongestants should be performed for superior visualization. Simple nasal polyps can cause constant nasal obstruction or have valve-like symptoms, where the sensation of airflow is better in one direction. Interestingly, symptom severity does not correlate with polyp size.[105] A nasal smear for eosinophilia can be performed to elucidate the etiology of polyposis; however a negative smear is not conclusive. Eosinophils in the nasal smear are elevated in acute, late and chronic phases of an allergic reaction.[106] Endoscopic nasal biopsy may be helpful to exclude more severe pathologies such as neoplasms and granulomatous disease.

Treatment of polyposis is important as it can lead to dramatic improvements in quality of life.[107,108] Treatment of nasal polyps

**Nasal Obstruction** 79

**Table 1:** Systemic etiologies of nasal obstruction

| Disease | Pathology | Presentation | Sinonasal symptoms | Diagnosis | Treatment |
|---|---|---|---|---|---|
| Granulomatosis with Polyangiitis Wegener's Granulomatosis | Idiopathic necrotizing upper + lower respiratory tract vasculitis | (1) Pulmonary sx's - hemoptysis, cough, dyspnea (2) Glomerulonephritis - hematuria, RBC casts (3) Systemic vasculitis - malaise, fever, arthralgia, myalgia | (1) Chronic sinusitis (2) Nasal deformity (3) Septal deviation (4) Epistaxis exam b/l swelling, crusting friable mucosa | (1) Antibodies (cANCA, PR3) (2) Pulmonary/nasal/renal biopsy | Systemic (1) Steroids (2) Cyclophosphamide, azathioprine, methotrexate Sinonasal (1) Hypertonic saline irrigation (2) Nasal debridement |
| Sarcoidosis | Noncaseating granulomas in the pulmonary system | (1) Systemic—fever, arthralgia, anorexic (2) Pulmonary—hemoptysis, dyspnea, chest pain, cough (3) Head & Neck—xerostomia, xerophthalmia, parotid enlargement | (1) Chronic sinusitis (2) Nasal crusting (3) Anosmia (4) Epistaxis (5) Lupus pernio (chronic indurated lesion, purple/raised) *hypertrophied friable mucosa, sub-mucosal nodules, and crusting* | (1) Histopathology (2) ^ACE levels (3) CXR → Bilateral hilar adenopathy | Systemic (1) Steroids (2) Cytotoxic, anti-malarial, and anti-tumor necrosis factor (TNF) agents Sinonasal (1) Topical steroids, low-dose systemic steroids, and nasal irrigation |

*Contd...*

*Contd...*

| Disease | Pathology | Presentation | Sinonasal symptoms | Diagnosis | Treatment |
|---|---|---|---|---|---|
| Churg-Strauss | Eosinophilic granulomatous vasculitis of small to medium sized vessels | (1) Systemic—constitutional symptoms. | (1) Allergic rhinitis (2) Nasal polyps (3) Asthma (4) Chronic sinusitis | (1) pANCA (2) ^ESR, ^CRP (3) Nasal biopsy (necrotizing vasculitis, extravascular granulomas, eosinophilia) | Systemic (1) High dose steroids Sinonasal (1) Symptomatic management. of allergic rhinitis (AR) (2) Surgical management of NP |
| T-Cell lymphoma | Abnormal T-cell proliferation | (1) Constitutional symptoms. (2) Cutaneous lesions | (1) Nasal obstruction (2) Epistaxis *Friable granulomatous tissue. Septal perforation* | (1) EBV+ (2) Nasal biopsy (NK markers and EBV DNA) | Systemic (1) Chemotherapy (2) Radiation Sinonasal (1) Symptomatic management. |

(RBC: Red blood cell; cANCA: Cytoplasmic antineutrophil cytoplasmic antibodies; ACE: Angiotensin converting enzyme; CXR: chest X-ray; pANCA: Perinuclear antineutrophil cytoplasmic antibodies; ESR: Erythrocyte sedimentation; CRP: C-reactive protein; EBV: Epstein–Barr virus; NK: Natural killer; DNA: deoxyribonucleic acid).

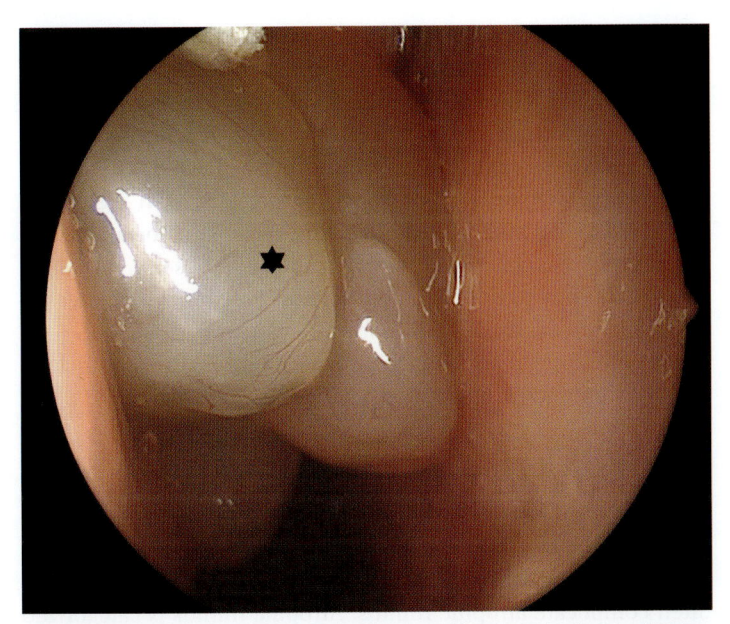

**Fig. 7:** Endoscopic view nasal polyposis. The asterisk marks the nasal polyp.

includes nasal lavage, topical steroids, a short course (2 weeks) of systemic steroids, a 12 week course of macrolide antibiotics in cases related to chronic rhinosinusitis, and antihistamines in allergic cases.[108-113] If these therapies fail to resolve symptoms within 4 weeks, a referral to an otolaryngologist is warranted for endoscopic examination. If medical management does improve symptoms, it is recommended to continue topical steroids. A trial of leukotriene antagonist may also improve chronic rhinosinusitis symptoms in some patients with polyposis, particularly those with aspirin sensitivity and asthma, and may be continued if efficacious.[114,115] Aspirin desensitization can be considered in patients with aspirin sensitivity related polyposis, but should be conducted by a specialist with close monitoring, as bronchospasm is a significant concern. If symptoms are not relieved with medical management, polypectomy can be considered, but polyp recurrence is common and continuation of medical management is recommended.[109]

## SUBJECTIVE NASAL OBSTRUCTION

The trigeminal nerve is responsible for determining the feeling of nasal obstruction by sensing nasal airflow patterns. Subjective complaints can occur both with and without an identifiable abnormality. Sensation of poor airflow in the absence of an identifiable anatomic or mucosal abnormality is seen in the normal physiologic nasal cycle and vasomotor rhinitis. The typical nasal cycle occurs due to cyclical changes in blood flow to the nasal mucosa mediated by fluctuations in sympathetic tone. This results in varying patency between the two nasal cavities. Vasomotor or idiopathic rhinitis is a diagnosis of exclusion. It presents with significant clear rhinorrhea and nasal obstruction often in association with temperature change, eating, smells and alcohol use. It is thought to be secondary to dysregulation of nasal function with increased parasympathetic stimulation without sympathetic balance. Two other syndromes that reflect subjective nasal obstruction include atrophic rhinitis and empty nose syndrome.

## Atrophic Rhinitis

Atrophic rhinitis is an uncommon syndrome characterized by atrophy of the mucosa, which presents with paradoxical nasal congestion. Bacterial colonization, thick nasal secretions, and sinusitis often complicate atrophic rhinitis. Atrophic rhinitis is categorized as either primary or secondary, however treatment remains similar. Nasal irrigation is helpful to remove crusts and a nasal lubricant may be applied to keep the nose moist. In some recalcitrant, cases, topical antibiotic lavage has been helpful.[116] Systemic antibiotics are needed periodically and should be guided by culture data. Vasoconstrictors and topical glucocorticoids should be avoided given compromised vasculature and immune defenses.[117]

### *Primary Atrophic Rhinitis*

Primary atrophic rhinitis predominantly affects young female patients from developing countries, typically with warmer climates.[118] It is thought that environmental factors, as illustrated by the increased incidence of industrial exposure in patients with atrophic rhinitis, and genetic predisposition play a role.[119,120] It has also been associated with colonization with *Klebsiella ozaenae*.[119] By definition, it occurs in people with no prior history of nasal trauma, surgery, radiation, or granulomatous disease. It typically presents with severe halitosis, nasal obstruction, anosmia, crusting, epistaxis, facial pain, sinusitis, and sleep disruption.[117] Patients will paradoxically report congestion because of the sensation of abnormal airflow. Nasal examination reveals thin, pale, shiny mucosa with crusts that may be bloody or purulent. Nasal endoscopy may reveal ulceration of nasal septum leading to perforation or even ulcerations of the lateral wall, resulting in a saddle nose deformity.[121] CT imaging may reveal mucosal atrophy of the middle and inferior turbinates and bony resorption with widening of the nasal cavity, mucosal thickening of the paranasal sinuses, and hypoplasia of the maxillary sinuses. Biopsy may be considered to ensure the absence of underlying inflammatory process, as in secondary atrophic rhinitis.

## Secondary Atrophic Rhinitis

Secondary atrophic rhinitis occurs as a result of prior trauma, surgery, radiation therapy, or inflammatory disease. Those secondary to prior sinus surgeries often suffer from stagnated mucus leading to bacterial superinfections and chronic rhinosinusitis, causing thick mucopurulent discharge. However, other patients with secondary atrophic rhinitis, particularly with sarcoidosis, will have dry noses with bloody scabs secondary to the destruction of the mucous glands by the disease process. Presenting complaints nearly always include nasal congestion, crusting and dryness, while other complaints include facial pain, epistaxis and anosmia. Anterior rhinoscopy reveals thin, edematous, erythematous mucosa. *P. aeruginosa* and *S. aureus* are the most common pathogens isolated for nasal swabs. Diagnostic criteria have been proposed, which include recurrent epistaxis, episodic anosmia, nasal purulence, crusting, chronic inflammatory condition, and two or more sinus surgeries. The presence of two or more criteria has 95% sensitivity and 77% specificity.[122,123] CT imaging is recommended, which may reveal diffuse mucosal changes and evidence of superinfection.

## Empty Nose Syndrome

Empty nose syndrome is an iatrogenic form of atrophic rhinitis that results from excess removal of the inferior turbinates. There is no consensus as to whether it is truly a different entity from secondary atrophic rhinitis and there is no consensus to define the syndrome, aside from widely patent nasal cavity with paradoxical nasal obstruction. It is thought that excess surgery leads to altered permeability of the mucosa and thus alters nasal airflow and humidification, which causes the symptoms of paradoxical nasal congestion.[124] It is thought that psychological factors play a role, as preoccupation with nasal symptoms, poor concentration, fatigue, irritability, anxiety, and depression are common.[125] Ipsilateral maxillary sinus opacification is a potential finding on radiography.[126] The moist cotton test, where a moistened piece of cotton is placed in the nasal cavity to redirect airflow, can be used to confirm the diagnosis if there is improvement. Conservative treatment with nasal hygiene and air humidification is preferred and should be used primarily. If conservative treatment fails and there is reversible pathology, a conservative surgical approach may be undertaken to reconstruct the turbinate.[124,125]

## APPROACH TO THE PATIENT WITH NASAL OBSTRUCTION

While there are a wide variety of causative factors for nasal obstruction, approaching the history and physical examination in a logical and stepwise fashion helps to facilitate the diagnosis. (A) Duration of symptoms and their progression is critical information, as it distinguishes between acute and chronic conditions. (B) Laterality is important as unilateral obstructions can suggest external and anatomic deficits such as septal deviation, polyps, or neoplasm versus bilateral nasal obstruction, which can occur secondary to allergies, sinusitis, or turbinate hypertrophy. (C) Presence or absence of rhinorrhea is especially important as purulent rhinorrhea can suggest acute sinusitis, and clear rhinorrhea can suggest vasomotor rhinitis. (D) Epistaxis in the setting of nasal obstruction can suggest the presence of a neoplasm. (E) Inquiries with respect to the environment and time of year can shed light on the role of allergies. (F) Loss of smell or hyposmia or even anosmia with nasal obstruction can occur due to polyps or secondary to allergies. (G) Facial/orbital pain and pressure can result from sinusitis, or the presence of a neoplasm. (H) History of facial trauma with nasal obstruction can suggest anatomic deficits such as septal deviation/perforation/hematoma, or nasal bone fracture. (I) In the setting of prior surgical or medical therapy once can consider scarring or synechiae formation, nasal tip deformity/valve collapse, or rhinitis medicamentosa. (J) Concomitant symptoms such as snoring and obstructive sleep apnea, excessive fatigue can suggest adenotonsillar hypertrophy. (K) Middle ear disease with nasal obstruction can be suspicious for nasopharyngeal neoplasm. (L) Smoking history also plays a role in nasal obstruction by affecting the action of cilia. (M) Systemic symptoms of conditions that affect the nose should also be considered especially in conditions such as hypothyroidism, Sjögren's syndrome, Wegener's granulomatosis, and obstructive sleep apnea-hypopnea syndrome (OSAHS).

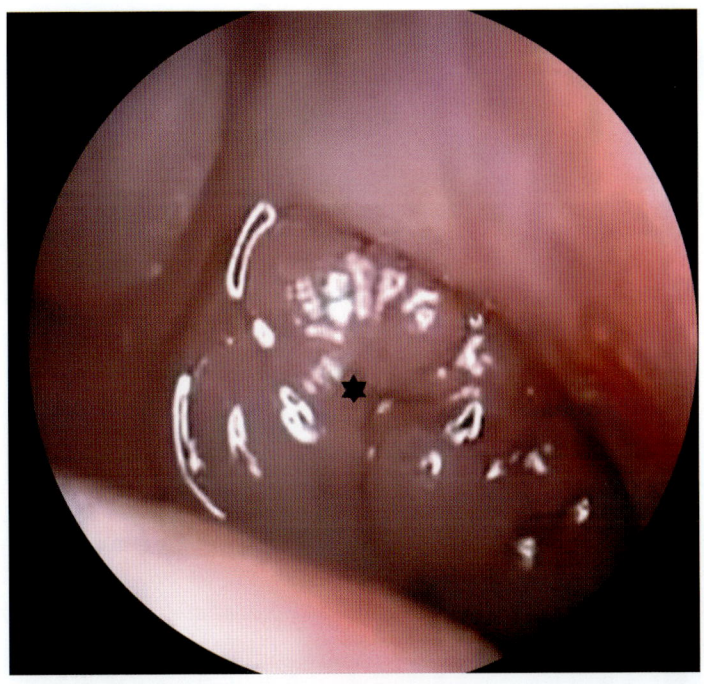

**Fig. 8:** Endoscopic view, adenoid hypertrophy, the nasopharynx is 100% obstructed. The asterisk marks the adenoid hypertrophy.

Upon completing the history a full head and neck examination is required to support the differential diagnosis formulated following the history. The most important portions of the physical for a complaint of nasal obstruction are the external and internal nasal examinations. The external nasal examination can demonstrate a deviated septum or valvular collapse on deep inspiration. The internal nasal examination facilitated by anterior rhinoscopy can help diagnose septal deviations, ITH, internal nasal valve collapse, and gross abnormalities in the form of polyps or masses. The examination of the middle ear can shed light whether there is an obstruction present at the end of the Eustachian tube orifice. Intraoral examination can demonstrate if there is adenotonsillar hypertrophy. Flexible fiberoptic nasal endoscopy and nasopharyngoscopy can clearly elucidate the presence of masses or polyps.

The diagnosis and treatment of nasal obstruction are contingent upon the cause. Table 2 lists symptoms, diagnostic tests, and treatment methodologies for common causes of nasal obstruction.

**Table 2:** Common causes of nasal obstruction and management

| Diagnosis | Symptoms | Test | Treatment |
|---|---|---|---|
| Septal deviation (Fig. 2) | Unilateral nasal obstruction | Computed tomography (CT) sinuses | Septoplasty |
| Septal perforation (Fig. 1) | Unilateral nasal obstruction | Rhinoscopy | Flaps—advancement, inferior turbinate |
| Septal hematoma | Pain in setting of recent trauma | Rhinoscopy | Incision and drainage, antibiotics |
| Septal abscess | (1) Pain<br>(2) Fever | Rhinoscopy | Incision and drainage, antibiotics |
| Nasal fracture | External deformity | (1) Direct inspection<br>(2) CT face | Reduction |
| Turbinate hypertrophy (Fig. 3) | Enlarged inferior turbinates | Rhinoscopy | (1) Medical → decongestants<br>(2) Surgical → turbinate resection, microdebrider reduction, turbinoplasty, radiofrequency, |
| Valvular collapse | Collapse with inspiration | (1) Observation<br>(2) Cottle test | (1) Supportive → à support strips, suspension<br>(2) Surgical → valvular reconstruction with grafts |
| Adenoid hypertrophy (Fig. 8) | (1) Unilateral/Bilateral<br>(2) Mouth breathing<br>(3) Snoring<br>(4) Dental crowding | (1) Oral examination<br>(2) Nasal endoscopy | Tonsillectomy/Adenoidectomy |
| OSAHS | (1) Thick palate<br>(2) Enlarged tonsils | Polysomnography | Uvulopalatopharyngoplasty |

*Contd...*

## Nasal Obstruction

*Contd...*

| Diagnosis | Symptoms | Test | Treatment |
|---|---|---|---|
| Choanal atresia (Fig. 4) | Unilateral/Bilateral Rhinorrhea | CT nasopharynx | Transpalatal repair |
| Polyps (Fig. 7) | (1) Unilateral/bilateral obstruction<br>(1) Impaired smell<br>(Asthma, aspirin-sensitive asthma (ASA) sensitivity) | Rhinoscopy | (1) Medical → steroids<br>(2) Surgical → polypectomy |
| Neoplasm (Figs. 5 and 6) | (1) Unilateral mass<br>(2) Impaired smell<br>(3) Epistaxis | (1) Nasal endoscopy<br>(2) CT<br>(3) MRI | Resection |
| Sinusitis (Figs. 9 and 10) | (1) Purulent mucous<br>(2) Pain/pressure over sinus/face | CT sinuses | Antibiotics |
| Vasomotor rhinitis | Clear mucous | By exclusion | Avoidance |
| Allergic rhinitis | (1) Hx of seasonal symptoms<br>(2) Boggy nasal mucosa | (1) Skin testing<br>(2) Radioallergosorbent test (RAST)<br>(3) Food allergen testing | (1) Avoidance<br>(2) Allergen desensitization<br>(3) Antihistamines<br>(4) Nasal steroids |
| Rhinitis medicamentosa | Clear mucous | History | (1) Steroids<br>(2) Avoiding decongestant sprays |
| Nasal foreign body | (1) Unilateral mass<br>(2) Purulent discharge | (1) Anterior rhinoscopy<br>(2) Nasal endoscopy | Removal of foreign body |

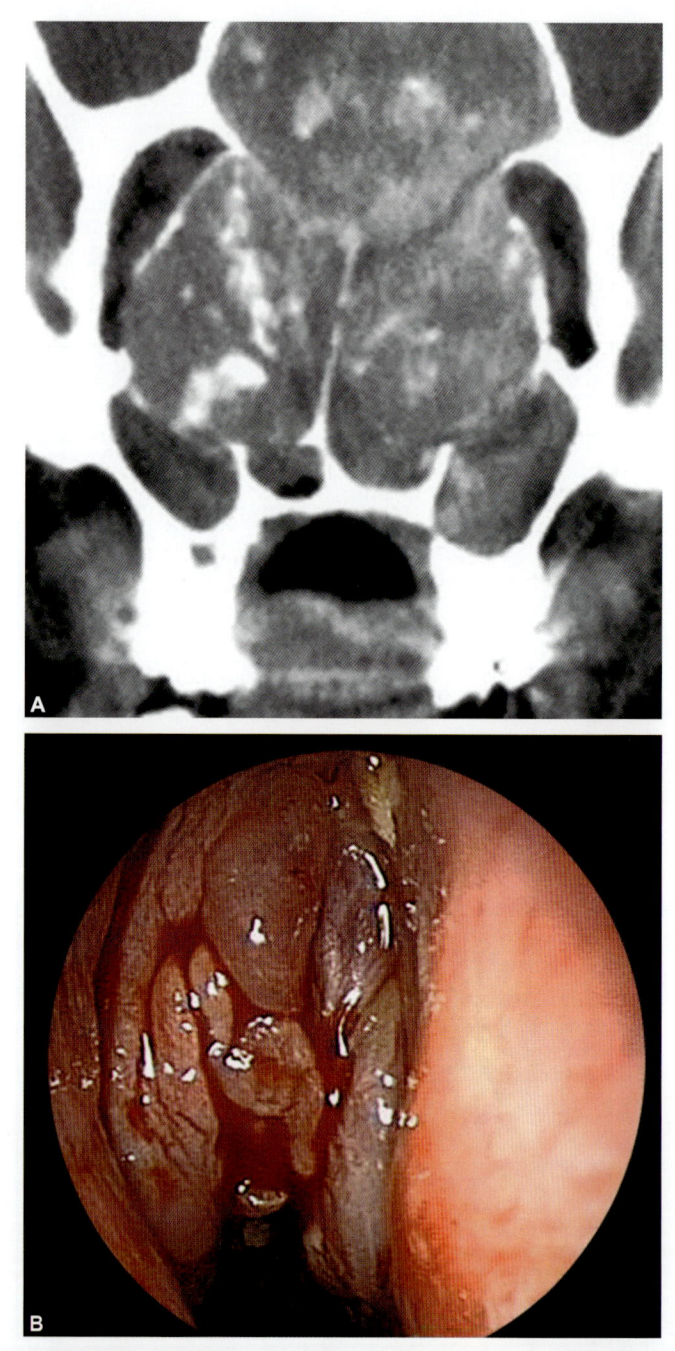

**Figs. 9A and B:** Invasive fungal sinusitis. (A) Coronal CT scan showing heterogeneous lesion; (B) Endoscopic view showing bleeding and inflammation.

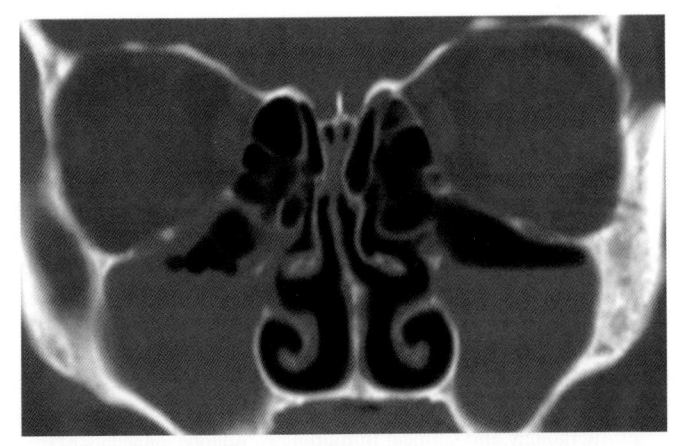

**Fig. 10:** Coronal computed tomography depicting bilateral acute maxillary sinusitis.

## REFERENCES

1. Leggett JE. Acute sinusitis. When—and when not—to prescribe antibiotics. Postgrad Med. 2004;115(1):13-9.
2. Stewart MG, Smith TL. Objective versus subjective outcomes assessment in rhinology. Am J Rhinol. 2005;19(5):529-35.
3. Meltzer EO. The prevalence and medical and economic impact of allergic rhinitis in the United States. J Allergy Clin Immunol. 1997;99(6 Pt 2):S805-28.
4. Skoner DP. Allergic rhinitis: definition, epidemiology, pathophysiology, detection, and diagnosis. J Allergy Clin Immunol. 2001;108 (1 Suppl):S2-8.
5. van Bavel J, Findlay SR, Hampel FC Jr, et al. Intranasal fluticasone propionate is more effective than terfenadine tablets for seasonal allergic rhinitis. Archives of internal medicine. 1994;154(23): 2699-704.
6. Kaszuba SM, Baroody FM, deTineo M, et al. Superiority of an intranasal corticosteroid compared with an oral antihistamine in the as-needed treatment of seasonal allergic rhinitis. Arch Intern Med. 2001;161(21):2581-7.
7. Weiner JM, Abramson MJ, Puy RM. Intranasal corticosteroids versus oral H1 receptor antagonists in allergic rhinitis: systematic review of randomised controlled trials. BMJ. 1998;317(7173):1624-9.
8. Allen DB, Meltzer EO, Lemanske RF Jr, et al. No growth suppression in children treated with the maximum recommended dose of fluticasone propionate aqueous nasal spray for one year. Allergy Asthma Proc. 2002;23(6):407-13.
9. Galant SP, Melamed IR, Nayak AS, et al. Lack of effect of fluticasone propionate aqueous nasal spray on the hypothalamic-pituitary-adrenal axis in 2- and 3-year-old patients. Pediatrics. 2003;112(1 Pt 1): 96-100.

10. Benninger MS, Ahmad N, Marple BF. The safety of intranasal steroids. Otolaryngol Head Neck Surg. 2003;129(6):739-50.
11. De Weck AL, Derer T, Bähre M. Investigation of the anti-allergic activity of azelastine on the immediate and late-phase reactions to allergens and histamine using telethermography. Clin Exp Allergy. 2000;30(2):283-7.
12. Berger W, Hampel F Jr, Bernstein J, et al. Impact of azelastine nasal spray on symptoms and quality of life compared with cetirizine oral tablets in patients with seasonal allergic rhinitis. Ann Allergy Asthma Immunol. 2006;97(3):375-81.
13. Lee TA, Pickard AS. Meta-analysis of azelastine nasal spray for the treatment of allergic rhinitis. Pharmacotherapy. 2007;27(6):852-9.
14. van Cauwenberge P, Bachert C, Passalacqua G, et al. Consensus statement on the treatment of allergic rhinitis. European Academy of Allergology and Clinical Immunology. Allergy. 2000;55(2):116-34.
15. Welsh PW, Stricker WE, Chu CP, et al. Efficacy of beclomethasone nasal solution, flunisolide, and cromolyn in relieving symptoms of ragweed allergy. Mayo Clinic proceedings. Mayo Clinic. 1987;62(2):125-34.
16. Orgel HA, Meltzer EO, Kemp JP, et al. Comparison of intranasal cromolyn sodium, 4%, and oral terfenadine for allergic rhinitis: symptoms, nasal cytology, nasal ciliary clearance, and rhinomanometry. Ann Allergy. 1991;66(3):237-44.
17. Hatton RC, Winterstein AG, McKelvey RP, et al. Efficacy and safety of oral phenylephrine: systematic review and meta-analysis. Ann Pharmacother. 2007;41(3):381-90.
18. Horak F, Zieglmayer P, Zieglmayer R, et al. A placebo-controlled study of the nasal decongestant effect of phenylephrine and pseudoephedrine in the Vienna Challenge Chamber. Ann Allergy Asthma Immunol. 2009;102(2):116-20.
19. Brozek JL, Bousquet J, Baena-Cagnani CE, et al. Allergic rhinitis and its impact on asthma (ARIA) guidelines: 2010 revision. J Allergy Clin Immunol. 2010;126(3):466-76.
20. Moscato G, Siracusa A. Rhinitis guidelines and implications for occupational rhinitis. Curr Opin Allergy Clin Immunol. 2009;9(2):110-5.
21. Philpott CM, El-Alami M, Murty GE. The effect of the steroid sex hormones on the nasal airway during the normal menstrual cycle. Clin Otolaryngol Allied Sci. 2004;29(2):138-42.
22. Bachert C. Persistent rhinitis - allergic or nonallergic? Allergy. 2004;59 Suppl 76:11-15; discussion 15.
23. Varghese M, Glaum MC, Lockey RF. Drug-induced rhinitis. Clin Exp Allergy. 2010;40(3):381-4.
24. Ellis AK, Keith PK. Nonallergic rhinitis with eosinophilia syndrome. Current allergy and asthma reports. 2006;6(3):215-20.
25. Meltzer EO, Hamilos DL. Rhinosinusitis diagnosis and management for the clinician: a synopsis of recent consensus guidelines. Mayo Clin Proc. 2011;86(5):427-43.

26. Seiberling KA, Grammer L, Kern RC. Chronic rhinosinusitis and superantigens. Otolaryngol Clin North Am. 2005;38(6):1215-36, ix.
27. Ponikau JU, Sherris DA, Kern EB, et al. The diagnosis and incidence of allergic fungal sinusitis. Mayo Clin Proc. 1999;74(9):877-84.
28. Chakrabarti A, Denning DW, Ferguson BJ, et al. Fungal rhinosinusitis: a categorization and definitional schema addressing current controversies. Laryngoscope. 2009;119(9):1809-18.
29. Wilson JF. In the clinic. Acute sinusitis. Ann Intern Med. 2010;153 (5):ITC31-15; quiz ITC316.
30. Meltzer EO, Hamilos DL, Hadley JA, et al. Rhinosinusitis: establishing definitions for clinical research and patient care. J Allergy Clin Immunol. 2004;114(6 Suppl):155-212.
31. Blomgren K, Alho OP, Ertama L, et al. Acute sinusitis: Finnish clinical practice guidelines. Scand J Infect Dis. 2005;37(4):245-50.
32. Benninger MS, Payne SC, Ferguson BJ, et al. Endoscopically directed middle meatal cultures versus maxillary sinus taps in acute bacterial maxillary rhinosinusitis: a meta-analysis. Otolaryngol Head Neck Surg. 2006;134(1):3-9.
33. Falagas ME, Karageorgopoulos DE, Grammatikos AP, et al. Effectiveness and safety of short vs. long duration of antibiotic therapy for acute bacterial sinusitis: a meta-analysis of randomized trials. Br J Clin Pharmacol. 2009;67(2):161-71.
34. Chim CS, Ma SY, Au WY, et al. Primary nasal natural killer cell lymphoma: long-term treatment outcome and relationship with the International Prognostic Index. Blood. 2004;103(1):216-21.
35. de Ferranti SD, Ioannidis JP, Lau J, et al. Are amoxycillin and folate inhibitors as effective as other antibiotics for acute sinusitis? A meta-analysis. BMJ. 1998;317(7159):632-7.
36. de Bock GH, Dekker FW, Stolk J, et al. Antimicrobial treatment in acute maxillary sinusitis: a meta-analysis. J Clin Epidemiol. 1997;50 (8):881-90.
37. Slavin RG, Spector SL, Bernstein IL, et al. The diagnosis and management of sinusitis: a practice parameter update. J Allergy Clin Immunol. 2005;116(6 Suppl):S13-47.
38. Kassel JC, King D, Spurling GK. Saline nasal irrigation for acute upper respiratory tract infections. Cochrane Database Syst Rev. 2010 (3):CD006821.
39. Zalmanovici Trestioreanu A, Yaphe J. Intranasal steroids for acute sinusitis. Cochrane Database Syst Rev. 2013;12:CD005149.
40. Braun JJ, Alabert JP, Michel FB, et al. Adjunct effect of loratadine in the treatment of acute sinusitis in patients with allergic rhinitis. Allergy. 1997;52(6):650-5.
41. Thomas M, Yawn BP, Price D, et al. EPOS Primary Care Guidelines: European Position Paper on the Primary Care Diagnosis and Management of Rhinosinusitis and Nasal Polyps 2007 - a summary. Prim Care Respir J. 2008;17(2):79-89.
42. Westerveld GJ, Voss HP, van der Hee RM, et al. Inhibition of nitric oxide synthase by nasal decongestants. Eur Respir J. 2000;16(3): 437-44.

43. Stringer SP, Mancuso AA, Avino AJ. Effect of a topical vasoconstrictor on computed tomography of paranasal sinus disease. Laryngoscope. 1993;103(1 Pt 1):6-9.
44. Inanli S, Ozturk O, Korkmaz M, et al. The effects of topical agents of fluticasone propionate, oxymetazoline, and 3% and 0.9% sodium chloride solutions on mucociliary clearance in the therapy of acute bacterial rhinosinusitis in vivo. Laryngoscope. 2002;112(2):320-5.
45. Caenen M, Hamels K, Deron P, et al. Comparison of decongestive capacity of xylometazoline and pseudoephedrine with rhinomanometry and MRI. Rhinology. 2005;43(3):205-9.
46. Graf PM. Rhinitis medicamentosa. Clin Allergy Immunol. 2007;19:295-304.
47. Rosenfeld RM, Andes D, Bhattacharyya N, et al. Clinical practice guideline: adult sinusitis. Otolaryngol Head Neck Surg. 2007;137(3 Suppl):S1-31.
48. Chow AW, Benninger MS, Brook I, et al. IDSA clinical practice guideline for acute bacterial rhinosinusitis in children and adults. Clin Infect Dis. 2012;54(8):e72-e112.
49. Subramanian HN, Schechtman KB, Hamilos DL. A retrospective analysis of treatment outcomes and time to relapse after intensive medical treatment for chronic sinusitis. Am J Rhinol. 2002;16(6):303-12.
50. Skorpinski EW, Vannelli PM, Yousef E, et al. Radiologic outcomes in children with chronic rhinosinusitis and ostiomeatal complex obstruction after medical management. Ann Allergy Asthma Immunol. 2008;100(6):529-32.
51. Ozturk F, Bakirtas A, Ileri F, et al. Efficacy and tolerability of systemic methylprednisolone in children and adolescents with chronic rhinosinusitis: a double-blind, placebo-controlled randomized trial. J Allergy Clin Immunol. 2011;128(2):348-52.
52. Lund VJ, Black JH, Szabo LZ, et al. Efficacy and tolerability of budesonide aqueous nasal spray in chronic rhinosinusitis patients. Rhinology. 2004;42(2):57-62.
53. Greene D. Total necrosis of the intranasal structures and soft palate as a result of nasal inhalation of crushed OxyContin. Ear Nose Throat J. 2005;84(8):512, 514, 516.
54. Baum ED, Boudousquie AC, Li S, et al. Sarcoidosis with nasal obstruction and septal perforation. Ear Nose Throat J. 1998;77(11):896-8, 900-892.
55. Avcin T, Silverman ED, Forte V, et al. Nasal septal perforation: a novel clinical manifestation of systemic juvenile idiopathic arthritis/adult onset Still's disease. J Rheumatol. 2005;32(12):2429-31.
56. Gandomi B, Bayat A, Kazemei T. Outcomes of septoplasty in young adults: the Nasal Obstruction Septoplasty Effectiveness study. Am J Otolaryngol. 2010;31(3):189-92.
57. Proctor DF. The upper airways. I. Nasal physiology and defense of the lungs. Am Rev Respir Dis. 1977;115(1):97-129.
58. Wittkopf M, Wittkopf J, Ries WR. The diagnosis and treatment of nasal valve collapse. Curr Opin Otolaryngol Head Neck Surg. 2008;16(1):10-13.

59. Belli E, Rendine G, Mazzone N. Concha bullosa: endoscopic treatment. J Craniofac Surg. 2009;20(4):1165-8.
60. Stallman JS, Lobo JN, Som PM. The incidence of concha bullosa and its relationship to nasal septal deviation and paranasal sinus disease. AJNR Am J Neuroradiol. 2004;25(9):1613-8.
61. Lam WW, Liang EY, Woo JK, et al. The etiological role of concha bullosa in chronic sinusitis. Eur Radiol. 1996;6(4):550-2.
62. Clark ST, Babin RW, Salazar J. The Incidence of Concha Bullosa and Its Relationship to Chronic Sinonasal Disease. Am J Rhinol. 1989;3(1):11-12.
63. Lathi A, Syed MM, Kalakoti P, et al. Clinico-pathological profile of sinonasal masses: a study from a tertiary care hospital of India. Acta Otorhinolaryngol Ital. 2011;31(6):372-7.
64. Bist SS, Varshney S, Baunthiyal V, et al. Clinico-pathological profile of sinonasal masses: An experience in tertiary care hospital of Uttarakhand. Natl J Maxillofac Surg. 2012;3(2):180-6.
65. Saettele M, Alexander A, Markovich B, et al. Congenital midline nasofrontal masses. Pediatr Radiol. 2012;42(9):1119-25.
66. Harley EH. Pediatric congenital nasal masses. Ear Nose Throat J. 1991;70(1):28-32.
67. Schlosser RJ, Faust RA, Phillips CD, et al. Three-dimensional computed tomography of congenital nasal anomalies. Int J Pediatr Otorhinolaryngol. 2002;65(2):125-31.
68. Hughes GB, Sharpino G, Hunt W, et al. Management of the congenital midline nasal mass: a review. Head Neck Surg. 1980;2(3):222-33.
69. MacEwen CJ, Young JD. Epiphora during the first year of life. Eye. 1991;5(Pt 5):596-600.
70. Hepler KM, Woodson GE, Kearns DB. Respiratory distress in the neonate. Sequela of a congenital dacryocystocele. Arch Otolaryngol Head Neck Surg. 1995;121(12):1423-5.
71. Adil E, Huntley C, Choudhary A, et al. Congenital nasal obstruction: clinical and radiologic review. Eur J Pediatr. 2012;171(4):641-50.
72. Wood JW, Casiano RR. Inverted papillomas and benign nonneoplastic lesions of the nasal cavity. Am J Rhinol Allergy. 2012;26(2):157-63.
73. Caruana SM, Zwiebel N, Cocker R, et al. p53 alteration and human papilloma virus infection in paranasal sinus cancer. Cancer. 1997;79(7):1320-8.
74. Lawson W, Patel ZM. The evolution of management for inverted papilloma: an analysis of 200 cases. Otolaryngol Head Neck Surg. 2009;140(3):330-5.
75. Martin H, Ehrlich HE, Abels JC. Juvenile Nasopharyngeal Angiofibroma. Ann Surg. 1948;127(3):513-36.
76. Park YW. Nasal granuloma gravidarum. Otolaryngol Head Neck Surg. 2002;126(5):591-2.
77. Zarrinneshan AA, Zapanta PE, Wall SJ. Nasal pyogenic granuloma. Otolaryngol Head Neck Surg. 2007;136(1):130-1.
78. Delbrouck C, Chamiec M, Hassid S, et al. Lobular capillary haemangioma of the nasal cavity during pregnancy. J Laryngology Otol. 2011;125(9):973-7.

79. Nanda VS. Common dermatoses. Part II. Am J Obstet Gynecol. 1996;174(4):1273-8.
80. Liebowitz D. Nasopharyngeal carcinoma: the Epstein-Barr virus association. Semin Oncol. 1994;21(3):376-81.
81. Yuan JM, Wang XL, Xiang YB, et al. Preserved foods in relation to risk of nasopharyngeal carcinoma in Shanghai, China. Int J Cancer. 2000;85(3):358-63.
82. Chien YC, Chen JY, Liu MY, et al. Serologic markers of Epstein-Barr virus infection and nasopharyngeal carcinoma in Taiwanese men. N Engl J Med. 2001;345(26):1877-82.
83. Lin JC, Wang WY, Chen KY, et al. Quantification of plasma Epstein-Barr virus DNA in patients with advanced nasopharyngeal carcinoma. N Engl J Med. 2004;350(24):2461-70.
84. Liao XB, Mao YP, Liu LZ, et al. How does magnetic resonance imaging influence staging according to AJCC staging system for nasopharyngeal carcinoma compared with computed tomography? Int J Radiat Oncol Biol Phys. 2008;72(5):1368-77.
85. Liu FY, Chang JT, Wang HM, et al. [18F]fluorodeoxyglucose positron emission tomography is more sensitive than skeletal scintigraphy for detecting bone metastasis in endemic nasopharyngeal carcinoma at initial staging. J Clin Oncol. 2006;24(4):599-604.
86. Bhattacharyya N. Cancer of the nasal cavity: survival and factors influencing prognosis. Arch Otolaryngol Head Neck Surg. 2002;128(9):1079-83.
87. Fornelli RA, Fedok FG, Wilson EP, et al. Squamous cell carcinoma of the anterior nasal cavity: a dual institution review. Otolaryngol Head Neck Surg. 2000;123(3):207-10.
88. Dulguerov P, Jacobsen MS, Allal AS, et al. Nasal and paranasal sinus carcinoma: are we making progress? A series of 220 patients and a systematic review. Cancer. 2001;92(12):3012-29.
89. Heffner DK, Hyams VJ, Hauck KW, et al. Low-grade adenocarcinoma of the nasal cavity and paranasal sinuses. Cancer. 1982;50(2):312-22.
90. Choussy O, Ferron C, Védrine PO, et al. Adenocarcinoma of Ethmoid: a GETTEC retrospective multicenter study of 418 cases. Laryngoscope. 2008;118(3):437-43.
91. Lupinetti AD, Roberts DB, Williams MD, et al. Sinonasal adenoid cystic carcinoma: the M. D. Anderson Cancer Center experience. Cancer. 2007;110(12):2726-31.
92. Dulguerov P, Allal AS, Calcaterra TC. Esthesioneuroblastoma: a meta-analysis and review. Lancet Oncol. 2001;2(11):683-90.
93. Mendenhall WM, Amdur RJ, Hinerman RW, et al. Head and neck mucosal melanoma. Am J Clin Oncol. 2005;28(6):626-30.
94. Clifton N, Harrison L, Bradley PJ, et al. Malignant melanoma of nasal cavity and paranasal sinuses: report of 24 patients and literature review. J Laryngol Otol. 2011;125(5):479-85.
95. Malowany MS, Chester B, Allerhand J. Isolation and microbiologic differentiation of Klebsiella rhinoscleromatis and Klebsiella ozaenae in cases of chronic rhinitis. Am J Clin Pathol. 1972;58(5):550-3.
96. Chan TV, Spiegel JH. Klebsiella rhinoscleromatis of the membranous nasal septum. J Laryngol Otol. 2007;121(10):998-1002.

97. Botelho-Nevers E, Gouriet F, Lepidi H, et al. Chronic nasal infection caused by Klebsiella rhinoscleromatis or Klebsiella ozaenae: two forgotten infectious diseases. Int J Infect Dis. 2007;11(5):423-9.
98. Shum TK, Whitaker CW, Meyer PR. Clinical update on rhinoscleroma. Laryngoscope. 1982;92(10 Pt 1):1149-53.
99. Fredricks DN, Jolley JA, Lepp PW, et al. Rhinosporidium seeberi: a human pathogen from a novel group of aquatic protistan parasites. Emerg Infect Dis. 2000;6(3):273-82.
100. Mendoza L, Taylor JW, Ajello L. The class mesomycetozoea: a heterogeneous group of microorganisms at the animal-fungal boundary. Annu Rev Microbiol. 2002;56:315-44.
101. Prabhu SM, Irodi A, Khiangte HL, et al. Imaging features of rhinosporidiosis on contrast CT. Indian J Radiol Imaging. 2013;23(3):212-8.
102. Job A, Venkateswaran S, Mathan M, et al. Medical therapy of rhinosporidiosis with dapsone. J Laryngol Otol. 1993;107(9):809-12.
103. Settipane GA. Epidemiology of nasal polyps. Allergy Asthma Proc. 1996;17(5):231-6.
104. Pawankar R. Nasal polyposis: an update: editorial review. Curr Opin Allergy Clin Immunol. 2003;3(1):1-6.
105. Johansson L, Akerlund A, Holmberg K, et al. Evaluation of methods for endoscopic staging of nasal polyposis. Acta Otolaryngol. 2000;120(1):72-6.
106. Godthelp T, Holm AF, Fokkens WJ, et al. Dynamics of nasal eosinophils in response to a nonnatural allergen challenge in patients with allergic rhinitis and control subjects: a biopsy and brush study. J Allergy Clin Immunol. 1996;97(3):800-11.
107. Uri N, Cohen-Kerem R, Barzilai G, et al. Functional endoscopic sinus surgery in the treatment of massive polyposis in asthmatic patients. J Laryngol Otol. 2002;116(3):185-9.
108. Ragab SM, Lund VJ, Scadding G. Evaluation of the medical and surgical treatment of chronic rhinosinusitis: a prospective, randomised, controlled trial. Laryngoscope. 2004;114(5):923-30.
109. Kalish L, Snidvongs K, Sivasubramaniam R, et al. Topical steroids for nasal polyps. Cochrane Database Syst Rev. 2012;12:CD006549.
110. Martinez-Devesa P, Patiar S. Oral steroids for nasal polyps. Cochrane Database Syst Rev. 2011;(7):CD005232.
111. Cervin A, Wallwork B. Efficacy and safety of long-term antibiotics (macrolides) for the treatment of chronic rhinosinusitis. Curr Allergy Asthma Rep. 2014;14(3):416.
112. Hissaria P, Smith W, Wormald PJ, et al. Short course of systemic corticosteroids in sinonasal polyposis: a double-blind, randomized, placebo-controlled trial with evaluation of outcome measures. J Allergy Clin Immunol. 2006;118(1):128-33.
113. Van Zele T, Gevaert P, Holtappels G, et al. Oral steroids and doxycycline: two different approaches to treat nasal polyps. J Allergy Clin Immunol. 2010;125(5):1069-76.e4.
114. Stewart RA, Ram B, Hamilton G, et al. Montelukast as an adjunct to oral and inhaled steroid therapy in chronic nasal polyposis. Otolaryngol Head Neck Surg. 2008;139(5):682-7.

115. Ragab S, Parikh A, Darby YC, et al. An open audit of montelukast, a leukotriene receptor antagonist, in nasal polyposis associated with asthma. Clin Exp Allergy. 2001;31(9):1385-91.
116. Leonard DW, Bolger WE. Topical antibiotic therapy for recalcitrant sinusitis. Laryngoscope. 1999;109(4):668-70.
117. Moore EJ, Kern EB. Atrophic rhinitis: a review of 242 cases. Am J Rhinol. 2001;15(6):355-61.
118. Dutt SN, Kameswaran M. The aetiology and management of atrophic rhinitis. J Laryngol Otol. 2005;119(11):843-52.
119. Han-Sen C. The ozena problem. Clinical analysis of atrophic rhinitis in 100 cases. Acta Otolaryngol. 1982;93(5-6):461-4.
120. Sibert JR, Barton RP. Dominant inheritance in a family with primary atrophic rhinitis. J Med Genet. 1980;17(1):39-40.
121. Kameswaran M. Fibre-optic endoscopy in atrophic rhinitis. J Laryngol Otol. 1991;105(12):1014-7.
122. deShazo RD, Stringer SP. Atrophic rhinosinusitis: progress toward explanation of an unsolved medical mystery. Curr Opin Allergy Clin Immunol. 2011;11(1):1-7.
123. Ly TH, deShazo RD, Olivier J, et al. Diagnostic criteria for atrophic rhinosinusitis. Am J Med. 2009;122(8):747-53.
124. Coste A, Dessi P, Serrano E. Empty nose syndrome. Eur Ann Otorhinolaryngol Head Neck Dis. 2012;129(2):93-7.
125. Chhabra N, Houser SM. The diagnosis and management of empty nose syndrome. Otolaryngol Clin North Am. 2009;42(2):311-30, ix.
126. Jang YJ, Kim JH, Song HY. Empty nose syndrome: radiologic findings and treatment outcomes of endonasal microplasty using cartilage implants. Laryngoscope. 2011;121(6):1308-12.

# Chapter 5

# Nasal Neoplasms

*Valeria Silva Merea, Ashutosh Kacker*

## INTRODUCTION

Sinonasal neoplasms are rare and their diagnosis may be delayed because their symptoms may mimic benign sinonasal disease. Prognosis improves with early detection. The most common presenting symptom is unilateral nasal obstruction. As tumors grow, however, they may lead to facial pain, epistaxis and other symptoms depending on the nearby structures they involve such as the orbit or the anterior cranial fossa. Unilateral nasal obstruction warrants a complete head and neck evaluation. Further workup with nasal endoscopy, imaging studies, and in most cases, histologic examination should also be considered.

The complete head and neck evaluation should include a careful examination of the nasal cavity with anterior rhinoscopy and nasal endoscopy. Oral cavity should be examined for any masses as tumors may invade into the maxilla. Any facial swelling or problems with the eyes and orbits need to be noted. A complete cranial nerve examination also provides important information on the extent of any potential masses. In addition, in any case of nasal obstruction, especially if unilateral, the ears need to be examined for serous otitis media. Finally, palpation of the neck looking for any enlarged lymph nodes should be performed. Upper jugulodigastric lymph nodes are commonly involved.

After a complete physical examination, imaging studies are used to define the extent and nature of the neoplasms. The main advantage of computed tomography (CT) over magnetic resonance imaging (MRI) is delineation of bony invasion, but MRI is superior at soft-tissue demarcation and distinguishing tumor from retained secretions. In addition, involvement of the anterior cranial fossa, skull base and orbit is best assessed with an MRI. If the diagnosis cannot be established with a physical examination and imaging, a biopsy may be necessary, but is not recommended if an angiofibroma is suspected because of the high risk of bleeding.

# BENIGN NASAL NEOPLASMS

## Osteoma

This is the most common benign neoplasm of the sinonasal tract. It is a slow growing tumor, slightly more common in males than females and usually diagnosed between the second and fifth decades of life. The frontal sinus is most commonly involved, followed by the ethmoid and maxillary sinuses, and rare sphenoid involvement. Of note, osteomas may be seen in people with Gardner's syndrome.

### Presentation

Most osteomas are asymptomatic, and are diagnosed incidentally on imaging studies performed for unrelated reasons. In some cases, osteomas interfere with sinus drainage and cause sinusitis and pain. In other cases and depending on location and pattern of growth, the presenting complaint may be aesthetic deformity. When osteomas grow toward the orbit, proptosis, orbital pain, epiphora or changes in visual acuity may be observed. Some osteomas extend into the anterior cranial fossa with a risk of cerebrospinal fluid leak, pneumocele, meningitis and brain abscess.

Endoscopic examination of the nasal cavity is usually normal when the lesions are deep into the paranasal cavities. However, in rare cases, a firm, mass covered by mucosa may be seen.

### Diagnosis

Osteomas are diagnosed by CT scans, and their appearance varies with the degree of mineralization of the bone within the lesion. Contrast is not necessary. MRI may be necessary in cases of bony erosion to better define the relationship between osteomas and adjacent soft tissues such as the meninges, brain and contents of the orbit.

### Treatment

For asymptomatic lesions that do not involve a critical structure, periodic imaging is usually the initial approach. In all other cases, surgery is performed. Most osteomas can be resected via a transnasal endoscopic approach. Tumors located on the lateral aspects of the frontal sinuses require an external approach.

Routine periodic imaging surveillance is usually not required because of the low risk of recurrence.

# Inverted Papillomas (Schneiderian Papilloma, Inverted Type)

This is the second most frequent benign tumor of the sinonasal tract, and it occurs most commonly in the lateral nasal wall, followed by the maxillary sinus. It is rarely found on the septum. Often, the exact site of origin cannot be assessed when tumors are large. Inverted papillomas tend to be unilateral, but may also present bilaterally. Men are more frequently affected than women. The incidence of these tumors ranges from 0.6 to 1.5 cases per 100,000 inhabitants per year. Human papilloma virus has been implicated in the etiology of these tumors. Studies have demonstrated the presence of serotypes 6, 11, 16 and 18. Squamous cell carcinoma (SCC) may be found within inverted papillomas; SCC prevalence is estimated between 3.4% and 9.7%.

## Presentation

These tumors usually present with unilateral nasal obstruction and watery rhinorrhea. Patients may also complain of facial pressure, headache or anosmia. Advanced lesions may present with epiphora, proptosis and diplopia. On examination, an inverted papilloma appears as a pale, polypoid lesion.

## Diagnosis

Histologic diagnosis is established by biopsy, usually performed under endoscopic guidance. Imaging studies are necessary to assess the extent of the tumor. MRI reveals a cerebriform-columnar pattern, and is better than a CT scan in differentiating tumor from mucosal changes or secretions.

## Treatment

Treatment of inverted papillomas is complete excision. This may be achieved through an open, endoscopic or combined approach. In order to achieve complete resection with an endoscopic approach, dissection of the mucosa along the subperiosteal plane and drilling of the underlying bone whenever necessary are required. Open approaches include medial maxillectomy through a lateral rhinotomy and midfacial degloving. Leaving a cavity that allows for wide access during endoscopic examinations facilitates follow-up examinations.

Postoperatively, nasal endoscopy is the primary method of tumor surveillance. However, imaging may be required to evaluate tumors when the original tumor site is not visible by endoscopy, when the patient is symptomatic or when a residual or recurrent lesion has been found.

## Juvenile Angiofibroma

Juvenile angiofibromas are highly vascular tumors that present in young adolescent males. Studies suggest that these lesions should be considered vascular malformations rather than tumors. Juvenile angiofibromas have a pathognomonic epicenter of origin in the pterygopalatine fossa, and spread from there.

### Presentation

Unilateral nasal obstruction and epistaxis are the most common symptoms at presentation. In advanced lesions, cheek swelling, proptosis or headache, which indicate involvement of the infratemporal fossa, orbit, or the cranial fossa respectively, may be seen. Nasal endoscopy reveals a smooth and hypervascularized lesion.

### Diagnosis

A characteristic hypervascular mass lesion in teenage boys with confirmation by CT or MRI provides the diagnosis. Imaging confirms the origin at the level of the pterygopalatine fossa, a characteristic anterior bowing of the posterior wall of the maxillary antrum, its hypervascularity after contrast enhancement and the pattern of growth. In-office biopsy is contraindicated when this tumor is suspected given high risk of hemorrhage (Figs. 1A and B).

### Treatment

Surgical resection is the mainstay of treatment. Open approaches have traditionally been used, but endoscopic approaches appear to be an alternative, and in some cases a combined approach is used. Preoperative angiography and embolization to decrease intraoperative bleeding is commonly performed. Low-dose radiation therapy is also an effective treatment modality for advanced or recurrent lesions not amenable to complete surgical resection.

Postoperative surveillance is performed with periodic endoscopic examinations and imaging studies. Contrast enhanced imaging is particularly important in the early detection of residual lesions because most of them tend to grow submucosally.

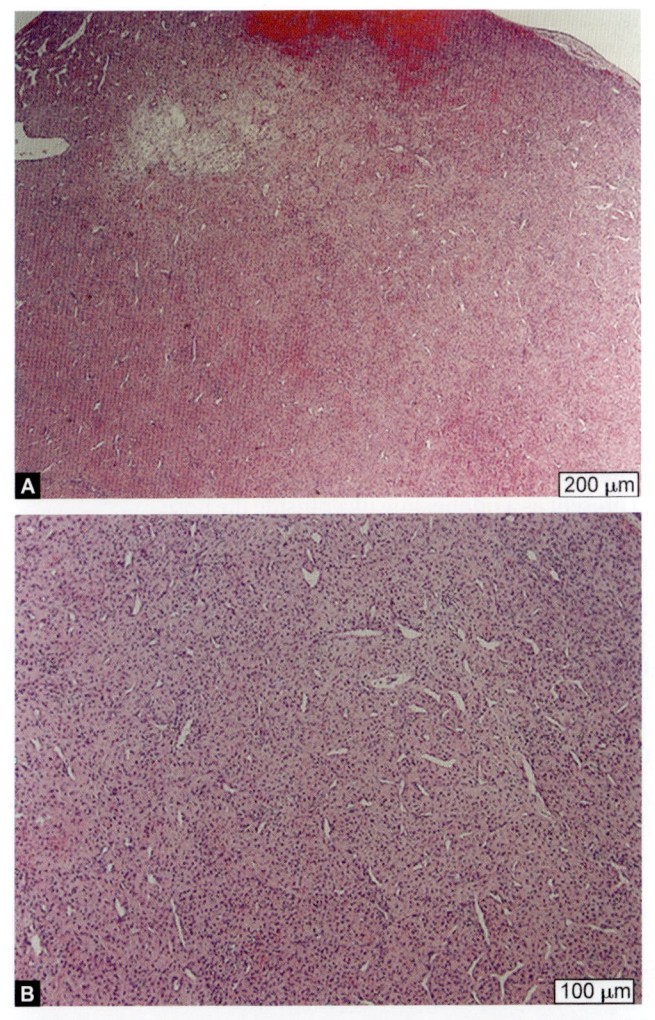

**Figs. 1A and B:** Pathology slides [Hematoxylin and Eosin (H&E) stain] of angiofibroma under low (A: 4x) and high (B: 10x) magnification. Biopsies are not done in the office because of high risk of bleeding. Figures by Theresa Scognamiglio, MD.

## MALIGNANT NASAL NEOPLASMS

The overall incidence of malignant sinonasal neoplasms is 0.556 cases per 100,000 population per year with a male:female ratio of 1.8:1, making these rare tumors. The most common malignant tumor is squamous cell carcinoma (SCC) followed by adenocarcinoma whereas the most common primary sites are the nasal cavity and maxillary sinuses. Prognostic factors generally include histological differentiation, tumor site, tumor stage, nodal involvement and treatment modality.

## Squamous Cell Carcinoma

This is the most common malignancy of the sinonasal cavity. They occur more commonly in males than females, and nickel workers appear to be at increased risk of developing these tumors.

### Presentation

Squamous cell carcinoma does not initially cause symptoms. As the mass grows, patients may experience nasal obstruction, discharge or epistaxis. These tumors may also have oral, ocular or facial involvement, leading to pain in the maxillary teeth, palate erosion, diplopia, proptosis and cheek swelling or paresthesias. They may also present as a nonhealing ulcer inside the nose.

### Diagnosis

Diagnosis is based on histologic analysis. Office biopsies may be obtained. SCC is hypointense on T2 images and heterogeneous with solid enhancement. CT scan demonstrates bony invasion in 80% of sinonasal SCCs (Fig. 2).

### Treatment

Treatment usually involves surgery and radiotherapy. Surgical procedures typically start with a maxillectomy, and may include orbital

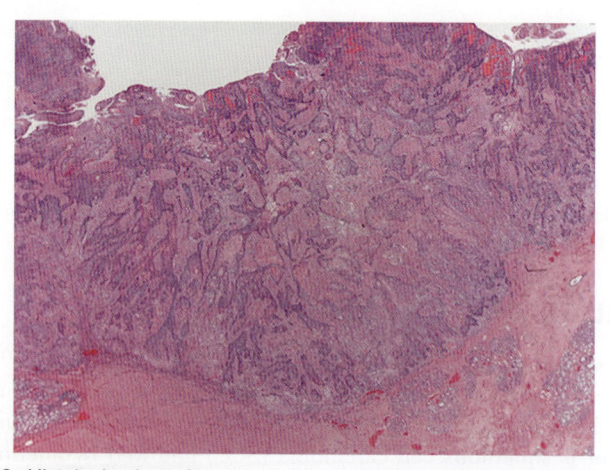

**Fig. 2:** Histologic view of squamous cell carcinoma (H&E stain). Figure by Theresa Scognamiglio, MD.

exenteration, infratemporal fossa dissection and craniofacial resection as necessary. Chemotherapy may also be used, especially for large tumors, and appears to improve locoregional control.

## Adenocarcinoma

This type of malignant tumors arises from the epithelial surface of the sinonasal mucosa. Hard wood dust and formaldehyde exposure have been found to increase the risk for developing sinonasal adenocarcinomas.

### Presentation

Nasal obstruction is the most common symptom at presentation. Tumors tend to arise from the ethmoid sinus.

### Diagnosis

Diagnosis is made by histologic analysis. Both degree of differentiation as well as tumor stage and extension impact prognosis. Mucinous and poorly differentiated carcinomas have been found to have shorter disease-free intervals and survival rates than well and moderately differentiated adenocarcinomas (Figs. 3A to C).

### Treatment

Surgical excision and postoperative radiation are typically used. Surgical approach varies with tumor site and extent, open and endoscopic approaches are used with similar results. An anterior craniofacial resection is used for advanced ethmoid cancers.

## Esthesioneuroblastoma

This type of tumor is also known as "olfactory neuroblastoma" because it arises from the olfactory epithelium within the nasal cavity, but it may invade the paranasal sinuses, orbit and skull base. It is a rare intranasal cancer, accounting for 1–6% of all intranasal malignancies.

### Presentation

Patients with esthesioneuroblastomas may present with nasal obstruction or discharge, epistaxis, sinus pain, visual changes, facial numbness or a neck mass. If tumor involves the frontal lobe, personality changes may be seen. Advanced local spread is common at presentation. Cervical lymph node metastases occur in up to a quarter of patients at presentation, whereas distant metastases have been reported in about 7% of patients.

## Diagnosis

Histologic diagnosis requires expertise and immunohistochemical investigations. Both CT and MRI are necessary as part of staging workup. CT gives information on bony erosion and MRI can provide more accurate detail of tumor extent into soft tissues including dura and brain. Recently, positron emission tomography (PET) scans have been recommended for staging.

## Treatment

Gold standard treatment is craniofacial resection, although endoscopic resection is increasingly being used. Resection with clear

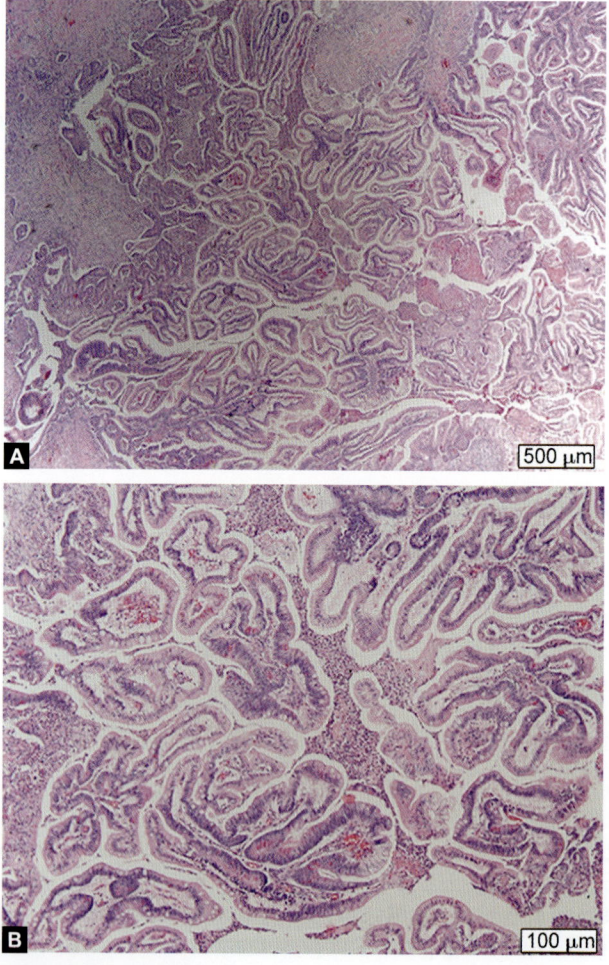

**Figs. 3A and B**

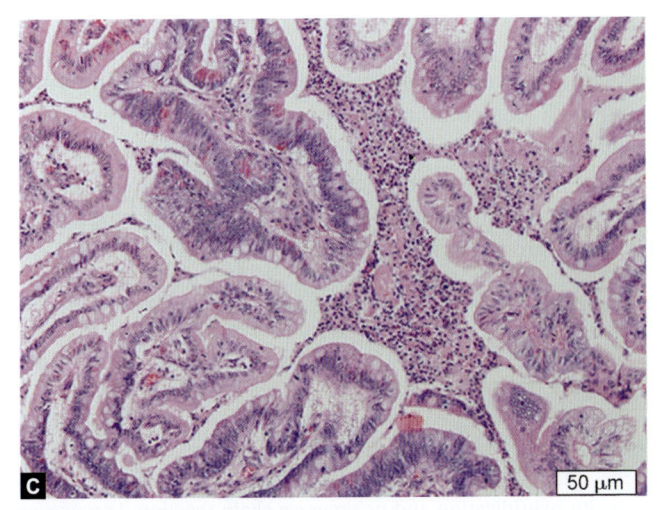

**Figs. 3A to C:** Pathology slides showing sinonasal adenocarcinoma under increasingly higher power. From A to C, 4x, 10x and 20x, respectively. Figures by Theresa Scognamiglio, MD

margins is essential. Postoperative concurrent chemotherapy and radiation therapy is also used as part of standard treatment. Elective treatment of the clinically negative neck is not usually done, but the neck should be included in follow-up imaging. Local and regional recurrence as well as distant metastases are common, and may occur years after presentation. No standardized protocols exist for surveillance, but serial MRI and endoscopic examinations have been recommended.

## Sinonasal Undifferentiated Carcinoma (SNUC)

This tumor is a rare and very aggressive malignant neoplasm with poor prognosis, characterized by rapid growth, locoregional recurrence and distant metastases. Tumors grow rapidly, and are prone to extensive local invasion into the sinuses, the orbit, and the brain.

### Presentation

Presentation varies with tumor extension. During early stages, findings are nonspecific. In case of orbital invasion, they may present with proptosis.

### Diagnosis

Tissue diagnosis requires microscopy and immunohistochemistry. Imaging studies of choice for staging are MRI and CT of the head and neck.

## Treatment

Treatment protocols are not well defined; however, a multimodality approach with combinations of surgery, radiation and chemotherapy is widely accepted. Total surgical resection is imperative, with craniofacial resection or endoscopic approaches, followed by concurrent chemoradiation. Even with combined multimodality approaches, prognosis remains poor.

## BIBLIOGRAPHY

1. Beham A, Beham-Schmid C, Regauer S, et al. Nasopharyngeal angiofibroma: true neoplasm or vascular malformation? Adv Anat Pathol. 2000;7(1):36-46.
2. Buchwald C, Franzmann MB, Jacobsen GK, et al. Human papillomavirus (HPV) in sinonasal papillomas: a study of 78 cases using in situ hybridization and polymerase chain reaction. Laryngoscope. 1995;105(1):66-71.
3. Buchwald C, Franzmann MB, Tos M. Sinonasal papillomas: a report of 82 cases in Copenhagen County, including a longitudinal epidemiological and clinical study. Laryngoscope. 1995;105(1):72-9.
4. Choussy O, Ferron C, Védrine PO, et al. Adenocarcinoma of Ethmoid: a GETTEC retrospective multicenter study of 418 cases. Laryngoscope. 2008;118(3):437-43.
5. Das S, Kirsch CF. Imaging of lumps and bumps in the nose: a review of sinonasal tumours. Cancer Imaging. 2005;5:167-77.
6. Enepekides DJ. Sinonasal undifferentiated carcinoma: an update. Curr Opin Otolaryngol Head Neck Surg. 2005;13(4):222-5.
7. Franchi A, Gallo O, Santucci M. Clinical relevance of the histological classification of sinonasal intestinal-type adenocarcinomas. Hum Pathol. 1999;30(10):1140-5.
8. Grégoire V, Lee N. Radiation therapy and management of the cervical lymph nodes and malignant skull base tumors. In: Flint PW, Haughey BH, Lund VJ, et al (Eds). Cummings Otolaryngology - Head & Neck Surgery. Philadelphia: Mosby Elsevier; 2010. pp. 1682-701. Print.
9. Harbo G, Grau C, Bundgaard T, et al. Cancer of the nasal cavity and paranasal sinuses. A clinico-pathological study of 277 patients. Acta Oncol. 1997;36(1):45-50.
10. Koka VN, Julieron M, Bourhis J, et al. Aesthesioneuroblastoma. J Laryngol Otol. 1998;112(7):628-33.
11. Lawson W, Patel ZM. The evolution of management for inverted papilloma: an analysis of 200 cases. Otolaryngol Head Neck Surg. 2009;140(3):330-5.
12. Lupinetti AD, Roberts DB, Williams MD, et al. Sinonasal adenoid cystic carcinoma: the M. D. Anderson Cancer Center experience. Cancer. 2007;110(12):2726-31.

13. Mandpe AH. Paranasal sinus neoplasms. In: Lalwani AK (Ed). Current Diagnosis & Treatment in Otolaryngology Head & Neck Surgery, 3rd edition. New York: McGraw Hill Medical; 2012. pp. 309-15.
14. Nicolai P, Castelnuovo P. Benign tumors of the sinonasal tract. In: Flint PW, Haughey BH, Lund VJ, et al (Eds). Cummings Otolaryngology - Head & Neck Surgery. Philadelphia: Mosby Elsevier; 2010. pp. 719-27. Print.
15. Rimmer J, Lund VJ, Beale T, et al. Olfactory neuroblastoma: a 35-year experience and suggested follow-up protocol. Laryngoscope. 2014;124(7):1542-9.
16. Suh JD, Chiu AG. What are the surveillance recommendations following resection of sinonasal inverted papilloma? Laryngoscope. 2014;124(9):1981-2.
17. Turner JH, Reh DD. Incidence and survival in patients with sinonasal cancer: a historical analysis of population-based data. Head Neck. 2012;34(6):877-85.
18. Van Gerven L, Jorissen M, Nuyts S, et al. Long-term follow-up of 44 patients with adenocarcinoma of the nasal cavity and sinuses primarily treated with endoscopic resection followed by radiotherapy. Head Neck. 2011;33(6):898-904.
19. Yoon BN, Batra PS, Citardi MJ, et al. Frontal sinus inverted papilloma: surgical strategy based on the site of attachment. Am J Rhinol Allergy. 2009;23(3):337-41.
20. Yoshida E, Aouad R, Fragoso R, et al. Improved clinical outcomes with multi-modality therapy for sinonasal undifferentiated carcinoma of the head and neck. Am J Otolaryngol. 2013;34(6):658-63.

# Chapter 6

# Epistaxis

*James Foshee, Alfred Marc Iloreta, Gurston G Nyquist, Marc R Rosen*

## EPIDEMIOLOGY

Epistaxis is a common condition that will occur in approximately 60% of individuals in the span of their lifetimes.[1] Epistaxis accounts for the second most common cause for emergency admission to otolaryngology services behind sore throat[2] and comprises nearly 0.5% of all emergency room visits in the United States.[3] Despite the high occurrence, only 6% of those experiencing an episode of epistaxis will present for medical treatment.[4]

Incidence is most common in pediatric patients, often younger than 10 years of age, and adults greater than 50 years of age.[1,5,6] In children, digital trauma, colloquially referred to as "nose-picking", is cited as the most common identifiable cause of epistaxis.[7] In adults, most cases are idiopathic in origin, with additional cases due to primary neoplasm, trauma to the head or face, or iatrogenic causes.[8,9] Conditions producing dryness of the nasal mucosa, such as heated indoor air in the winter and nasal cannula for oxygen delivery, also contribute to the incidence of epistaxis.[10] This is exacerbated by deviations in the nasal septum where disruption of nasal airflow causes dry air to contact the same spot along the anterior septum. Additional causes may be secondary to systemic conditions, such as coagulopathies (e.g. Von Willebrand disease or hemophilia disorders), hereditary hemorrhagic telangiectasia, viral or bacterial rhinosinusitis, or anticoagulant medication usage, such as Warfarin.[10] The incidence of epistaxis is also higher in hypertensive patients. Nasal insufflation of illicit drugs, such as cocaine, can also cause epistaxis, either through direct trauma to the nasal mucosa, or due to the vasoactive properties of the drug itself.[11] While most cases of epistaxis are idiopathic in origin,[12] a complete medical history can help rule-out other causal factors. Identifying and correcting possible causes of epistaxis can facilitate more effective management.

Severity of epistaxis episodes can range from fairly innocuous to life threatening, requiring immediate medical attention. Deaths due to epistaxis are rare, but do occur.[10] Mortality typically arises from airway obstruction,[2] therefore proper maintenance of a patent airway is paramount in the management of epistaxis.

## ANATOMY

Due to the direct apposition of the nasal vasculature to the underlying bony and cartilaginous structures of the nasal cavity walls, there is little extracellular support for the vessels. As such, the vasculature of the nose is particularly susceptible to physical trauma or irritation, such as drying of the mucosa.

Epistaxis can be divided into anterior and posterior bleeds using the ostium of the maxillary sinus as a division line. Anterior bleeds generally occur anterior to the ostium.[13] This region of the nasal septum contains a series of anastomoses between branches of the internal and external carotid arteries. Among these arteries are terminal branches of the sphenopalatine and greater palatine arteries (branches of the internal maxillary artery), anterior and posterior ethmoidal arteries (branches of the ophthalmic artery), and the superior labial artery (terminal branch of the facial artery). Together, these vessels form an arterial watershed area referred to as Kiesselbach's plexus (Fig. 1).[14]

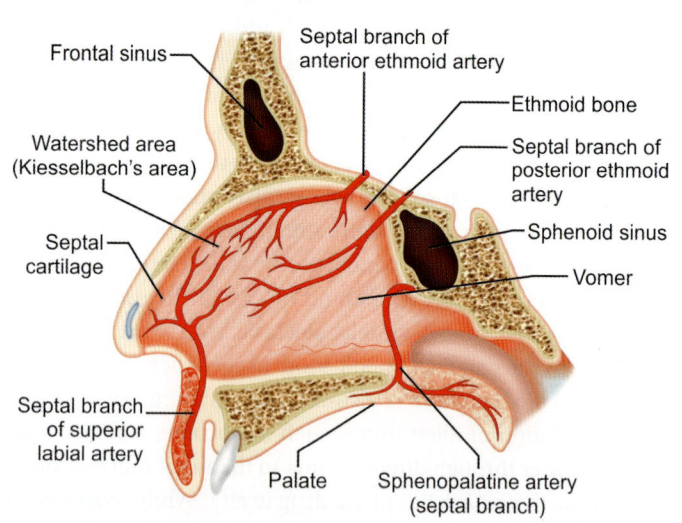

**Fig. 1:** Kiesselbach's plexus: Series of anastomoses between branches of the internal and external carotid arteries. Among these arteries are terminal branches of the sphenopalatine and greater palatine arteries (branches of the internal maxillary artery), anterior and posterior ethmoidal arteries (branches of the ophthalmic artery), and the superior labial artery (terminal branch of the facial artery).

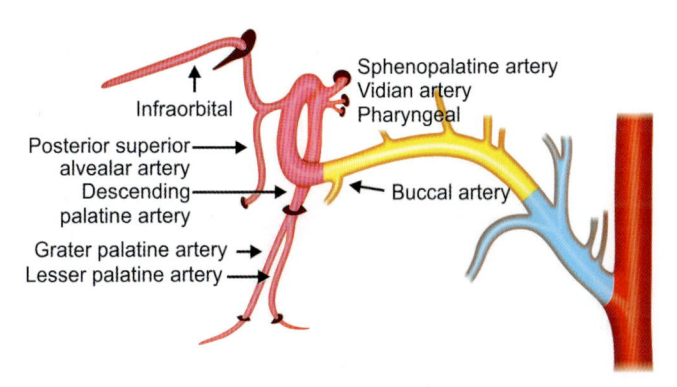

**Fig. 2:** The sphenopalatine artery that supplies the posterior blood supply via the sphenopalatine foramen in a posterolateral-superior location, where it branches to form septal and conchal branches.[14] In 12% of patients, the sphenopalatine artery enters the posterior nasal cavity via an alternative foramen.

Posterior bleeds commonly arise posterior to the ostium of the maxillary sinus from branches of the sphenopalatine artery, a branch of the external carotid. This artery enters the nasal cavity via the sphenopalatine foramen in a posterolateral-superior location, where it branches to form septal and conchal branches (Fig.2).[14] In 12% of patients, the sphenopalatine artery enters the posterior nasal cavity via an alternative foramen. Thus, care should be taken when performing endoscopic ligation on patients with posterior epistaxis to address variations in anatomy.[15] Posterior epistaxis can also originate from the descending palatine arteries or the internal carotid.[16] Posterior bleeds are more likely to require emergency medical treatment due to voluminous hemorrhage.

Bleeding from the lateral nasal cavity wall, via the ethmoidal arteries (Fig. 3), is possible, but not common. Epistaxis originating in this region is often due to facial trauma or iatrogenic injury related to sinus surgery.[8]

## MANAGEMENT

As with any emergent patient, management of the ABC's (airway, breathing, circulation) should be a primary priority. Maintaining a patent airway is most important in epistaxis, as it is possible for the nasal hemorrhage to pass into the oropharynx and block the airway.[17] Hypovolemia due to blood loss is not common,[8] although severe bleeds may require particular vigilance in monitoring proper volume status.

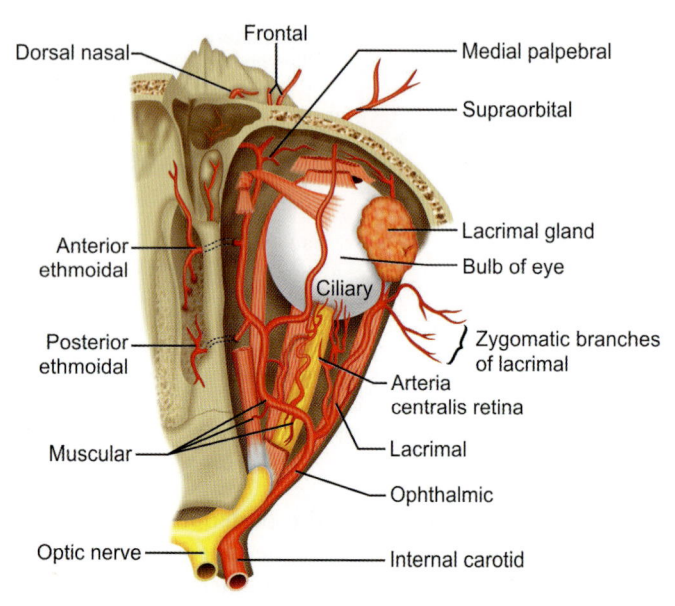

**Fig. 3:** The anterior ethmoid artery originates from the ophthalmic artery which is a direct branch of the internal carotid artery. This supplies the anterior aspect of the lateral nasal wall as the ethmoidal cells and portions of the septum.

Greater than 90% of epistaxis episodes will arise from the vessels of Kiesselbach's plexus, thus classified as anterior bleeds.[18] Only about 5% of cases are due to posterior epistaxis,[19,20] although these posterior bleeds are often more severe.[21] Management of the bleed will vary depending on the location of origin of epistaxis and the severity of the hemorrhage. Localization of nasal hemorrhages can be performed through a nasal speculum, generally for anterior epistaxis, or nasal endoscopy for more posteriorly located bleeds.[6,21]

## ANTERIOR EPISTAXIS

Anterior epistaxis generally does not require medical treatment and will often resolve spontaneously or respond well to simple first-aid measures.[8,17] Sustained digital pressure applied to the anterior nasal ala while the patient leans forward can often resolve anterior epistaxis.[22] Having the patient lean forward can prevent compromise of the airway by the nasal hemorrhaging.[23] Addition of a topical vasoconstrictor like oxymetazoline after blowing clot from the nose can also be useful in promoting hemostasis.[23]

## Nasal Packing

For anterior bleeds not resolving spontaneously or with applied pressure, nasal packing is the mainstay of treatment.[8,24] Packing traditionally involves the introduction of ribbon gauze (Fig. 4) coated in petroleum jelly (Vaseline) to apply mechanical pressure to the site of hemorrhage from within the nasal cavity. Ribbon gauze packing is introduced to the nasal cavity in a pleated fashion, taking special caution to avoid causing further damage to the nasal mucosa.[10] Alternatively, specially designed packing materials, such as the Rapid Rhinonasal packing (Fig. 5; ArthroCare Corp., Austin, TX, USA) or the Merocel nasal tampon pack (Fig. 6; Medtronic ENT, Jacksonville, FL, USA), has become the preferred method of applying pressure as the risk of nasal trauma is less and simplifies the packing procedure.[8] Nasal packing for anterior epistaxes has reported success rates as high as 85%.[25] The selection of packing material

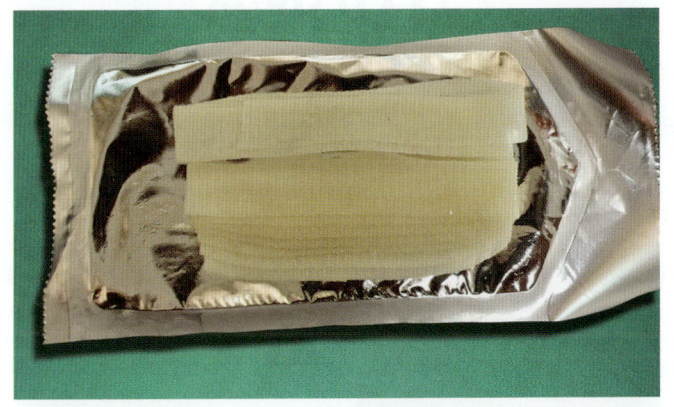

**Fig. 4:** 0.5 inch × 72 inch fine mesh gauze impregnated with petroleum jelly.

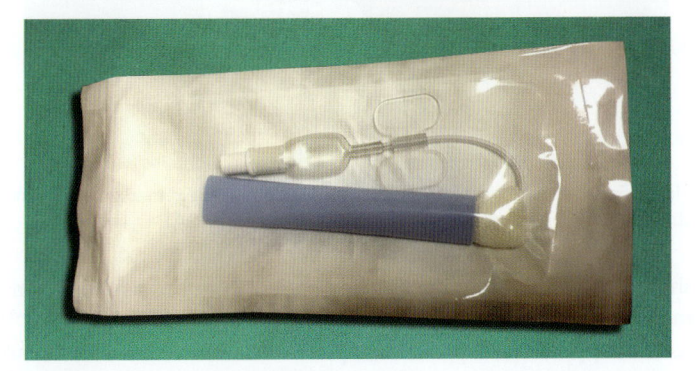

**Fig. 5:** Rapid Rhinonasal packing.

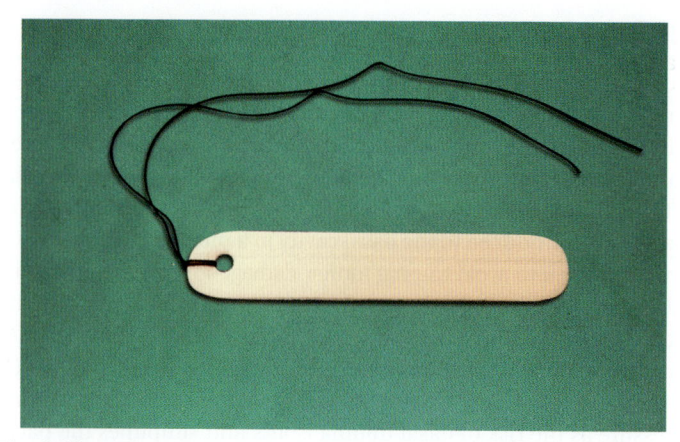

**Fig. 6:** Merocel nasal tampon (Medtronic ENT, Jacksonville, FL, USA).

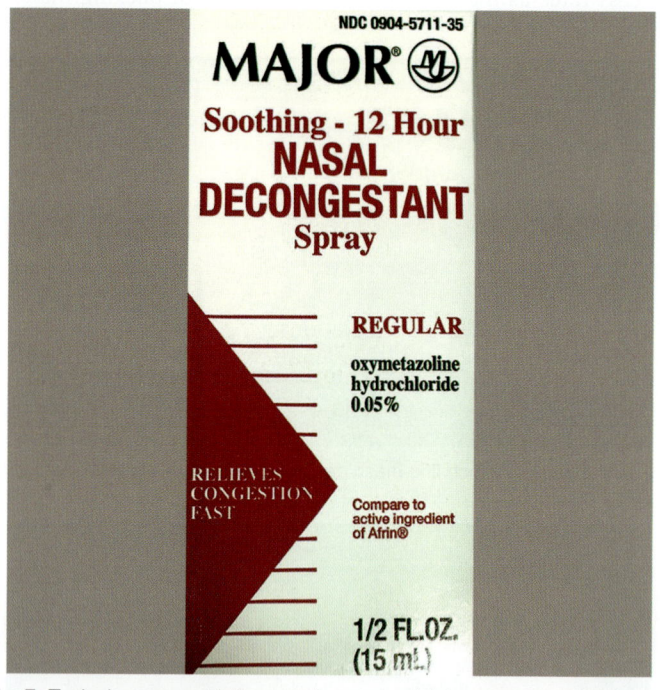

**Fig. 7:** Topical vasoconstrictive nasal spray containing oxymetazoline hydrochloride 0.05% (Major Pharmaceuticals, Livonia, MI, USA).

should revolve around maximizing patient comfort, as most common forms of packing have demonstrated comparable efficacy.[26-28] As with applied nasal pressure, topical vasoconstrictors (Fig. 7) can be applied to control bleeding and promote patient comfort.

Packing materials in the nasal cavity can cause significant patient discomfort, as well as adverse reactions, such as dyspnea, nasal infection, pressure necrosis of the nasal septum or ala, hypoxia, or toxic shock syndrome.[24,29,30] Toxic shock is a reaction to exotoxins released from Gram-positive *Staphylococcus aureus*, possibly introduced during the nasal packing procedure. Symptoms include nausea, vomiting, hypotension, mucosal hyperemia and elevated temperatures.[10] Prophylactic antibiotics[31] as well as topical antibiotic treatment after removal of packing may be helpful in preventing toxic shock development in epistaxis patients.[16] The use of specifically manufactured nasal packing materials, such as Merocel, can also reduce the incidence of toxic shock syndrome.[32]

In patients where the area of active hemorrhage is clearly identified, or the patient will not tolerate packing, or those experiencing treatment failure, then cauterization is effective in managing anterior bleeds.[25,33] While some evidence recommends cauterization as a secondary treatment for patient's that are refractory to nasal packing, other evidence suggests cauterization as an effective first-line treatment for epistaxis.[13,34,35] As both nasal packing and cauterization have demonstrated efficacy in treating epistaxes, selection of either procedure should depend on the provider's expertise and the patient's preference.

## Cauterization

Chemical or electrical cauterizations are both useful when the origin of hemorrhage is readily identifiable in the anterior nasal cavity.[16,34] Local anesthesia that includes topical application of a vasoconstrictor (like phenylephrine) and anesthetic agent (like ponticaine) is necessary for patient comfort. Depending on the cauterization technique, a local injection of lidocaine with epinephrine may be prudent. The provider should aspirate before the injection to ensure that the injection is not intravascular. Chemical cauterization with silver nitrate (Fig. 8), applied with an applicator, is an effective method to promote hemostasis,[2,36] with success rates reportedly as high as 94% in cases of anterior epistaxis.[13] Cauterization can be applied to both the origin of the bleed and the immediately surrounding nasal mucosa to reduce the risk of recurrence.[36] Dark discolorations of the mucosa (nasal "tattooing") and septal perforations are possible side-effects of the procedure.[2,15] Electrocautery can be useful when bleeding is too rapid for chemical cauterization (Fig. 9),[8] and it does not carry the same risk of discoloration, although septal perforation is also possible.[16]

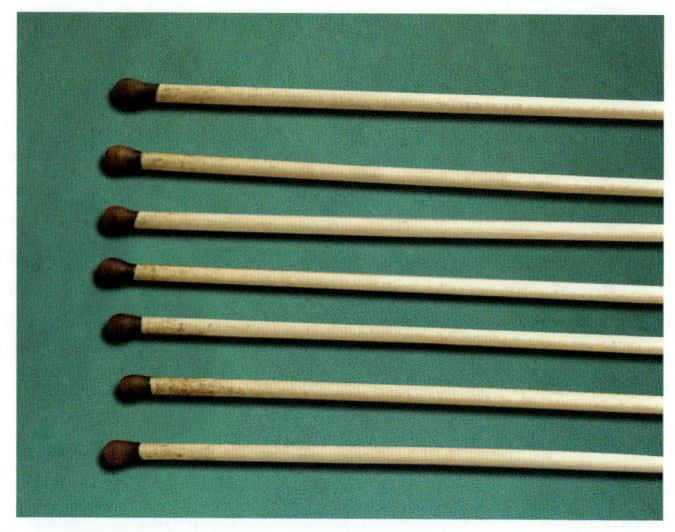

**Fig. 8:** Silver nitrate chemical cauterization sticks.

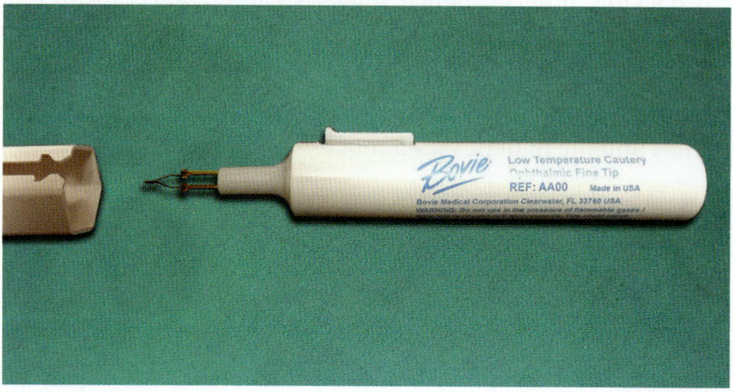

**Fig. 9:** Low temperature portable thermal cautery (Bovie Medical Corporation, Clearwater, FL, USA).

## Thrombogenic Agents

An additional treatment alternative involves the use of thrombogenic agents applied to the nasal cavity to promote hemostasis (Figs. 10A and B). Some evidence, albeit in small trials, suggests thrombogenic agents, such as Floseal (a recombinant thrombin gel manufactured by Baxter Healthcare Corp, Deerfield, IL, USA), can be more effective in resolving bleeds, preventing recurrence, and may be more comfortable to patients when compared to nasal packing alone.[27,37] Thrombogenic agents present a less invasive alternative to surgery, and may be an effective treatment in the control of recurrent or refractory epistaxis not responding to nasal packing alone.

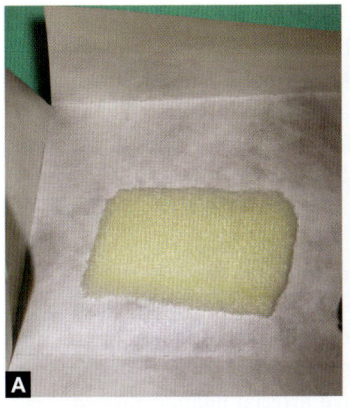

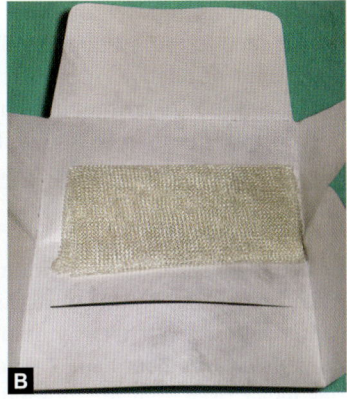

**Figs. 10A and B:** Oxidized regenerated cellulose manufactured by Ethicon Sarl, Neuchatel, Switzerland.

## POSTERIOR EPISTAXIS

Epistaxes originating posterior to the maxillary sinus ostium (representing approximately 5% of epistaxes[38]) are typically more voluminous and may require more invasive management techniques than anterior epistaxes.[15] These cases of epistaxis are thought to originate primarily from branches of the sphenopalatine artery.[15]

### Nasal Packing

Initial treatment for a posterior nasal hemorrhage often involves nasal packing.[13,39] In addition to the packs used for anterior bleeds, the specially designed inflatable Rhino Rocket balloon (Shippert Medical Technologies Corp., Centennial, CO, USA), Merocel, and the Epistat nasal catheter (Medtronic Xomed Surgical, Minneapolis, MN USA) are available.[8] Foley catheters, commonly found in most medical practices or hospitals, may also be used if other packing materials are unavailable. The catheter is advanced through the nasal cavity into the oropharynx, inflated, and then retracted to lodge in the posterior nasal cavity.[10] Double-sided packing, where both the affected and unaffected nasal cavities are packed, can apply increased mechanical pressure on the site of epistaxes, although this can cause a decrease in oxygen saturation and patients should be monitored with telemetry and continuous pulse oximetry.[40]

Similar to anterior nasal packing, posterior packing carries risks of dysphagia, dyspnea, pressure necrosis of the nasal septum, infection, significant discomfort or pain,[41] as well as hypoxia.[42,43] Posterior packing has been suggested to increase vagal tone, thus inducing bradycardia and hypotension in some patients.[44] Admittance to the hospital for observance is recommended with placement of bilateral nasal packs, formal posterior packing like an Epistat, and if cardiopulmonary symptoms are suspected. In addition to the potential side-effects, nasal packing for posterior epistaxis has failure rates reportedly between 26% and 54%.[34,45]

## Cauterization

Posterior epistaxis not responding to nasal packing may be candidates for other more invasive procedures. Direct endoscopic cauterization is an effective method when the origin of the hemorrhage is clearly identified.[8] Cauterization is less invasive and carries fewer risks than the alternative arterial ligation procedures,[46] although septal perforation is still possible.

## Endoscopic Arterial Ligation

For intractable posterior bleeds, or those posterior epistaxes refractory to nasal packing, endoscopic sphenopalatine arterial ligation (ESPAL) is indicated,[41,47,48] with reported success rates between 75% and 100%.[49-52] Side-effects for ESPAL are relatively minor, and can include decreased lacrimation, paresthesias of the nose or palate, and nasal crusting, although septal perforations and necrosis are also possible.[34,48,53] A more formal internal maxillary artery ligation can also be performed via an endoscopic transmaxillary approach or a caldwell-luc incision in cases refractory to ESPAL. These surgical approaches do carry the inherent risks associated with general anesthesia.

## Endovascular Embolization

An additional method for control of refractory posterior epistaxis is endovascular embolization.[54-56] First performed in 1974,[57] the current usage of embolization procedures for epistaxis is on the rise.[58] Angiography is typically performed prior to the procedure to localize the location of the vessel lesion,[58] followed by advancement of a transfemoral catheter and introduction of embolizing materials into either the sphenopalatine or facial arteries. Anatomically variable anastomoses between the external and internal carotid arteries may exist;[55,59] therefore, caution should be taken during embolization to avoid dislodging pre-existing atherosclerotic plaques which may enter the internal carotid circulation causing cerebrovascular accidents (CVAs).[58] Embolization of the ethmoidal arteries cannot be performed as these are branches of the ophthalmic artery, and there is significant risk for blindness and stroke.

Reported success rates for endovascular embolization in the management of posterior epistaxis range from 79% to 96%.[59,60] The procedure does, however, carry significant risks. Possible risks of embolization in the treatment of epistaxis include arterial dissection, facial skin necrosis, paresthesias, blindness, ophthalmoplegia, and most importantly, an increased risk for CVAs, namely ischemic stroke.[54,55,61] Although studies have either been inconclusive or have not indicated an increased mortality risk when compared to arterial ligation,[51,58,62] it is well-accepted that embolization has a statistically significant increased risk for CVAs, such as stroke,[58,63] with a reported risk near 1%.[58] Due to the extreme invasiveness of the procedure, as well as the potential risks, it would be prudent to restrict the usage of endovascular embolization to cases of epistaxis refractory to other, less invasive methods of treatment.

Patients presenting with facial trauma, particularly to the naso-ethmoid orbital region[35] can have bleeds of the lateral nasal cavity wall, often originating from the anterior ethmoidal artery.[2] These patients typically do not respond to basic treatments, such as packing, and will often require surgery.[64,65] In this setting and refractory cases of epistaxis not controlled with packing, cauterization and ESPAL procedures, then endoscopic or open anterior and posterior ethmoid artery ligation is indicated.

Patients with systemic causes for epistaxis are challenging to control until the underlying cause is addressed. Coagulopathies, anticoagulant usage, or primary neoplasms are frequent causes recurrent epistaxis.[8,15] Management of the underlying potential causes will facilitate more successful treatment of epistaxis episodes in these patients. Often this requires stopping medications, use of medications to reverse coagulopathies and transfusion of blood products. Consultation by medical specialists proves critical in this setting.

## CONCLUSION

Epistaxis is an extremely common problem encountered by otolaryngologists. Although several varying treatment algorithms have been proposed,[16,20,34,66] most advocate a step-wise approach to the management of epistaxis based on the location and severity of the bleeds, as well as the response to treatment and possibility of recurrence. Initial localization of the origin of the bleed is necessary, as location can guide treatment options. Practitioners should also be wary of systemic conditions that can predispose patients to epistaxis. Severe bleeds, such as those originating in the posterior nasal cavity, or those refractory to more conservative treatments like nasal packing, may necessitate more invasive management procedures, such as surgical ligation or endovascular embolization. All of the procedures mentioned in this review are not without substantial risks; therefore determination of management decisions should be made on a case-by-case basis. More conservative management is recommended initially, as most cases of epistaxis will resolve either spontaneously or with minimal intervention. An incremental increase in invasive treatments will typically resolve most cases of epistaxis.

## REFERENCES

1. Pollice PA, Yoder MG. Epistaxis: a retrospective review of hospitalized patients. Otolaryngol Head Neck Surg. 1997;117(1):49-53.
2. Barnes ML, Spielmann PM, White PS. Epistaxis: a contemporary evidence based approach. Otolaryngol Clin North Am. 2012;45(5): 1005-17.
3. Rudmik L, Smith TL. Management of intractable spontaneous epistaxis. Am J Rhinol Allergy. 2012;26(1):55-60.
4. Small M, Murray JA, Maran AG. A study of patients with epistaxis requiring admission to hospital. Health Bull (Edinb). 1982;40(1):20-9.
5. Petruson B. Epistaxis. A clinical study with special reference to fibrinolysis. Acta Otolaryngol Suppl. 1974;317:1-73.
6. Sengupta A, Maity K, Ghosh D, et al. A study on role of nasal endoscopy for diagnosis and management of epistaxis. J Indian Med Assoc. 2010;108(9):597-8, 600-1.
7. Gilyoma JM, Chalya PL. Etiological profile and treatment outcome of epistaxis at a tertiary care hospital in Northwestern Tanzania: a prospective review of 104 cases. BMC Ear Nose Throat Disord. 2011;11:8.
8. Shukla PA, Chan N, Duffis EJ, et al. Current treatment strategies for epistaxis: a multidisciplinary approach. J Neurointerv Surg. 2013;5(2): 151-6.
9. Varshney S, Saxena RK. Epistaxis: A retrospective clinical study. Indian J Otolaryngol Head Neck Surg. 2005;57(2):125-9.
10. Kasperek ZA, Pollock GF. Epistaxis: an overview. Emerg Med Clin North Am. 2013;31(2):443-54.
11. Jewers WM, Rawal YB, Allen CM, et al. Palatal perforation associated with intranasal prescription narcotic abuse. Oral Surg Oral Med Oral Pathol Oral Radiol Endod. 2005;99(5):594-7.
12. Walker TW, Macfarlane TV, McGarry GW. The epidemiology and chronobiology of epistaxis: an investigation of Scottish hospital admissions 1995-2004. Clin Otolaryngol. 2007;32(5):361-5.
13. Supriya M, Shakeel M, Veitch D, et al. Epistaxis: prospective evaluation of bleeding site and its impact on patient outcome. J Laryngol Otol. 2010;124(7):744-9.
14. Koh E, Frazzini VI, Kagetsu NJ. Epistaxis: vascular anatomy, origins, and endovascular treatment. AJR Am J Roentgenol. 2000;174(3): 845-51.

15. Douglas R, Wormald PJ. Update on epistaxis. Curr Opin Otolaryngol Head Neck Surg. 2007;15(3):180-3.
16. Hudson JW. Epistaxis: diagnosis and treatment. J Oral Maxillofac Surg. 2006;64(6):995.
17. Middleton PM. Epistaxis. Emerg Med Australas. 2004;16(5-6):428-40.
18. Alvi A, Joyner-Triplett N. Acute epistaxis. How to spot the source and stop the flow. Postgrad Med. 1996;99(5):83-90, 94-6.
19. Viducich, RA, Blanda MP, Gerson LW. Posterior epistaxis: clinical features and acute complications. Ann Emerg Med. 1995;25(5):592-6.
20. Spielmann PM, Barnes ML, White PS. Controversies in the specialist management of adult epistaxis: an evidence-based review. Clin Otolaryngol. 2012;37(5):382-9.
21. Supriya, M, Shakeel M, Veitch D, et al. Epistaxis: prospective evaluation of bleeding site and its impact on patient outcome. J Laryngol Otol. 2010;124(7):744-9.
22. Perretta LJ, Denslow BL, Brown CG. Emergency evaluation and management of epistaxis. Emerg Med Clin North Am. 1987;5(2):265-77.
23. Kucik CJ, Clenney T. Management of epistaxis. Am Fam Physician. 2005;71(2):305-11.
24. Goddard JC, Reiter ER. Inpatient management of epistaxis: outcomes and cost. Otolaryngol Head Neck Surg. 2005;132(5):707-12.
25. Kotecha, B, Fowler S, Harkness P, et al. Management of epistaxis: a national survey. Ann R Coll Surg Engl. 1996;78(5):444-6.
26. Corbridge RJ, Djazaeri B, Hellier WP, et al. A prospective randomized controlled trial comparing the use of merocel nasal tampons and BIPP in the control of acute epistaxis. Clin Otolaryngol Allied Sci. 1995;20(4):305-7.
27. Mathiasen RA, Cruz RM. Prospective, randomized, controlled clinical trial of a novel matrix hemostatic sealant in patients with acute anterior epistaxis. Laryngoscope. 2005;115(5):899-902.
28. Singer AJ, Blanda M, Cronin K, et al. Comparison of nasal tampons for the treatment of epistaxis in the emergency department: a randomized controlled trial. Ann Emerg Med. 2005;45(2):134-9.
29. de Vries N, van der Baan S. Toxic shock syndrome after nasal surgery: is prevention possible? A case report and review of the literature. Rhinology. 1989;27(2):125-8.
30. Schaitkin B, Strauss M, Houck JR. Epistaxis: medical versus surgical therapy: a comparison of efficacy, complications, and economic considerations. Laryngoscope. 1987;97(12):1392-6.
31. Hull HF, Mann JM, Sands CJ, et al. Toxic shock syndrome related to nasal packing. Arch Otolaryngol. 1983;109(9):624-6.
32. Breda SD, Jacobs JB, Lebowitz AS, et al. Toxic shock syndrome in nasal surgery: a physiochemical and microbiologic evaluation of Merocel and NuGauze nasal packing. Laryngoscope. 1987;97(12):1388-91.
33. Toner JG, Walby AP. Comparison of electro and chemical cautery in the treatment of anterior epistaxis. J Laryngol Otol. 1990;104(8): 617-8.
34. Shargorodsky J, Bleier BS, Holbrook EH, et al. Outcomes analysis in epistaxis management: development of a therapeutic algorithm. Otolaryngol Head Neck Surg. 2013;149(3):390-8.

35. Spielmann PM, Barnes ML, White PS. Controversies in the specialist management of adult epistaxis: an evidence-based review. Clin Otolaryngol. 2012;37(5):382-9.
36. Hanif J, Tasca RA, Frosh A, et al. Silver nitrate: histological effects of cautery on epithelial surfaces with varying contact times. Clin Otolaryngol Allied Sci. 2003;28(4):368-70.
37. Côté D, Barber B, Diamond C, et al. FloSeal hemostatic matrix in persistent epistaxis: prospective clinical trial. J Otolaryngol Head Neck Surg. 2010;39(3):304-8.
38. Tan LK, Calhoun KH. Epistaxis. Med Clin North Am. 1999;83(1):43-56.
39. McGarry GW, Aitken D. Intranasal balloon catheters: how do they work? Clin Otolaryngol Allied Sci. 1991;16(4):388-92.
40. Ogretmenoglu O, Yilmaz T, Rahimi K, et al. The effect on arterial blood gases and heart rate of bilateral nasal packing. Eur Arch Otorhinolaryngol. 2002;259(2):63-6.
41. Klotz DA, Winkle MR, Richmon J, et al. Surgical management of posterior epistaxis: a changing paradigm. Laryngoscope. 2002;112(9):1577-82.
42. Lin YT, Orkin LR. Arterial hypoxemia in patients with anterior and posterior nasal packings. Laryngoscope. 1979;89(1):140-4.
43. Hady MR, Kodeira KZ, Nasef AH. The effect of nasal packing on arterial blood gases and acid-base balance and its clinical importance. J Laryngol Otol. 1983;97(7):599-604.
44. Cassisi NJ, Biller HF, Ogura JH. Changes in arterial oxygen tension and pulmonary mechanics with the use of posterior packing in epistaxis: a preliminary report. Laryngoscope. 1971;81(8):1261-6.
45. Schaitkin B, Strauss M, Houck JR. Epistaxis: medical versus surgical therapy: a comparison of efficacy, complications, and economic considerations. Laryngoscope. 1987;97(12):1392-6.
46. Elwany S, Abdel-Fatah H. Endoscopic control of posterior epistaxis. J Laryngol Otol. 1996;110(5):432-4.
47. Asanau A, Timoshenko AP, Vercherin P, et al. Sphenopalatine and anterior ethmoidal artery ligation for severe epistaxis. Ann Otol Rhinol Laryngol. 2009;118(9):639-44.
48. Snyderman CH, Goldman SA, Carrau RL, et al. Endoscopic sphenopalatine artery ligation is an effective method of treatment for posterior epistaxis. Am J Rhinol. 1999;13(2):137-40.
49. Kumar S, Shetty A, Rockey J, et al. Contemporary surgical treatment of epistaxis. What is the evidence for sphenopalatine artery ligation? Clin Otolaryngol Allied Sci. 2003;28(4):360-3.
50. Nouraei SA, Maani T, Hajioff D, et al. Outcome of endoscopic sphenopalatine artery occlusion for intractable epistaxis: a 10-year experience. Laryngoscope. 2007;117(8):1452-6.
51. Elahi MM, Parnes LS, Fox AJ, et al. Therapeutic embolization in the treatment of intractable epistaxis. Arch Otolaryngol Head Neck Surg. 1995;121(1):65-9.
52. Abdelkader M, Leong SC, White PS. Endoscopic control of the sphenopalatine artery for epistaxis: long-term results. J Laryngol Otol. 2007;121(8):759-62.

53. Moorthy R, Anand R, Prior M, et al. Inferior turbinate necrosis following endoscopic sphenopalatine artery ligation. Otolaryngol Head Neck Surg. 2003;129(1):159-60.
54. Vokes DE, McIvor NP, Wattie WJ, et al. Endovascular treatment of epistaxis. ANZ J Surg. 2004;74(9):751-3.
55. Willems PW, Farb RI, Agid R. Endovascular treatment of epistaxis. AJNR Am J Neuroradiol. 2009;30(9):1637-45.
56. Risley J, Mann K, Jones NS. The role of embolisation in ENT: an update. J Laryngol Otol. 2012;126(3):228-35.
57. Sokoloff J, Wickbom I, McDonald D, et al. Therapeutic percutaneous embolization in intractable epistaxis. Radiology. 1974;111(2):285-7.
58. Brinjikji W, Kallmes DF, Cloft HJ. Trends in epistaxis embolization in the United States: a study of the Nationwide Inpatient Sample 2003-2010. J Vasc Interv Radiol. 2013;24(7):969-73.
59. Tseng EY, Narducci CA, Willing SJ, et al. Angiographic embolization for epistaxis: a review of 114 cases. Laryngoscope. 1998;108(4 Pt 1):615-9.
60. Smith TP. Embolization in the external carotid artery. J Vasc Interv Radiol. 2006;17(12):1897-912; quiz 1913.
61. Kagetsu NJ, Berenstein A, Choi IS. Interventional radiology of the extracranial head and neck. Cardiovasc Intervent Radiol. 1991;14(6):325-33.
62. Strong EB, Bell DA, Johnson LP, et al. Intractable epistaxis: transantral ligation vs. embolization: efficacy review and cost analysis. Otolaryngol Head Neck Surg. 1995;113(6):674-8.
63. Sadri M, Midwinter K, Ahmed A, et al. Assessment of safety and efficacy of arterial embolisation in the management of intractable epistaxis. Eur Arch Otorhinolaryngol. 2006;263(6):560-6.
64. Woolford TJ, Jones NS. Endoscopic ligation of anterior ethmoidal artery in treatment of epistaxis. J Laryngol Otol. 2000;114(11):858-60.
65. Camp AA, Dutton JM, Caldarelli DD. Endoscopic transnasal transethmoid ligation of the anterior ethmoid artery. Am J Rhinol Allergy. 2009;23(2):200-2.
66. Schlosser RJ. Clinical practice. Epistaxis. N Engl J Med. 2009;360(8):784-9.

# Chapter 7

# Common Nasal and Sinus Pathologies in Children

*Karin PQ Oomen, Ashutosh Kacker*

## SINUSITIS

Pediatric sinusitis remains one of the most common diseases of childhood. Rhinosinusitis can be considered a spectrum of disease characterized by concurrent inflammatory and infectious processes that affect the nasal passages and the contiguous paranasal sinuses.[1-3] Children average six to eight colds per year, with 0.5–5% developing sinus infections. It is commonly agreed that if common cold symptoms are not improving by 7–10 days, a sinus infection should be considered.[4] Because common viral upper respiratory infections and acute sinusitis can be difficult to distinguish clinically, acute episodes of sinusitis have traditionally been defined as the persistence of signs and symptoms beyond 10 days, or the concomitant occurrence of related complications, such as orbital abscess or meningitis. The definition of chronic rhinosinusitis (CRS) has largely been accepted as the persistence of characteristic signs and symptoms beyond 12 weeks.

Along with the nasal passages, the paranasal sinuses filter, warm, and humidify inspired air. They may also play a role in reducing the overall weight of the human skull. Sinuses grow in size and shape throughout childhood. The frontal sinuses are the last to fully develop, and generally reach adult size by puberty. The primary common factor in the pathophysiology of sinus disease is an inciting event or process, which leads to inflammation and obstruction of sinus ostia. This leads to stasis of secretions and impaired ventilation of the sinus. Absorption of oxygen and development of negative pressure within the sinus then ensues. This draws intranasal and nasopharyngeal contents (including bacteria) into the affected sinus. Bacterial infection has long been considered a key component of CRS, and the pathogens found in children are generally similar to those in adults. The common isolates associated with CRS include those found in acute sinusitis (*Streptococcus pneumoniae*, *Moraxella catarrhalis* and *Haemophilus influenzae*) as well as

*Staphylococcus aureus*, Pseudomonas and anaerobes. The role of fungi has also been proposed, but remains controversial.[5] Local or anatomic factors include direct sinus obstruction caused by anatomic abnormalities, such as the presence of concha bullosa, septal deviation, nasal polyposis, trauma and foreign bodies. Conditions contributing to mucosal inflammation and secondary obstruction include upper respiratory tract infection, allergy, immunodeficiencies, ciliary dyskinesia, cystic fibrosis and gastroesophageal reflux disease (GERD). GERD in particular is known to be prevalent in children with CRS.[6] A retrospective study has shown a significant decrease in the need for sinus surgery among children on antireflux therapy.[7] In addition to allergens, environmental irritants, such as air pollutants or tobacco smoke may occasionally play a role in chronic mucosal inflammation.

The symptoms of acute or chronic sinusitis in children are different from those in adult patients and include persistent cough, and prolonged rhinorrhea and/or postnasal drip, congestion, low-grade fever, irritability, and even behavioral difficulties. Headache, a prominent symptom in adults, is less commonly present in children. A nasal foreign body should be considered in children with a history of prolonged unilateral rhinorrhea with a foul odor reported by parents.

When sinusitis is suspected, a full head and neck examination is warranted. Anterior rhinoscopy will show mucosal erythema and irritation, thickened nasal mucous, and sometimes frank purulent drainage. When nasal polyps are present, cystic fibrosis should be considered as a possible diagnosis, and further workup in this area is recommended. Fiberoptic nasal endoscopy may reveal purulent drainage in the middle meatus coming from the maxillary and ethmoid sinuses. In many children, an enlarged adenoid will be present. The diagnosis of sinusitis remains primarily a clinical one. Most otolaryngologists advocate computed tomography (CT) scans of the sinuses only when deciding on surgical intervention (Figs. 1 and 2).

The most effective method of treating acute sinusitis remains subject of debate. Most clinicians feel that if the symptoms have persisted for 7–10 days the infection should be treated with antibiotics for at least 14 days. However, the natural history of acute rhinosinusitis is that close to 65% of cases will spontaneously resolve.[8] The American Academy of Pediatrics has set forth treatment guidelines based on the available literature or group consensus.[9] For young children with acute rhinosinusitis, amoxicillin is recommended for those who do not attend daycare and have not recently received antibiotics.

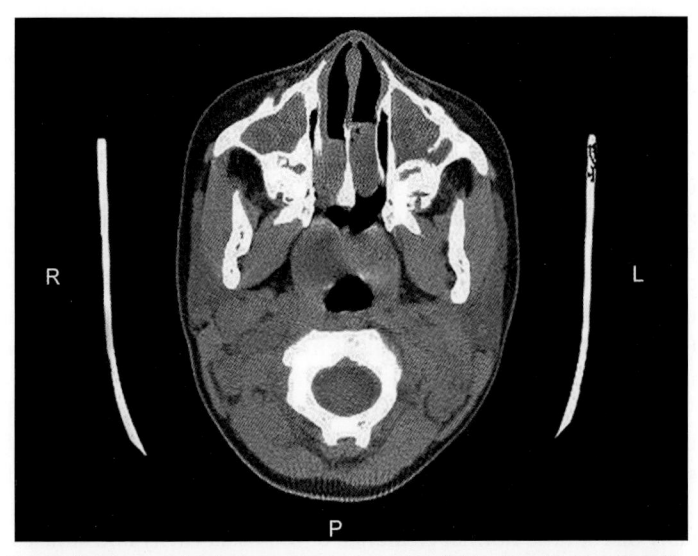

**Fig. 1:** Axial computed tomography image of pediatric chronic rhinosinusitis.

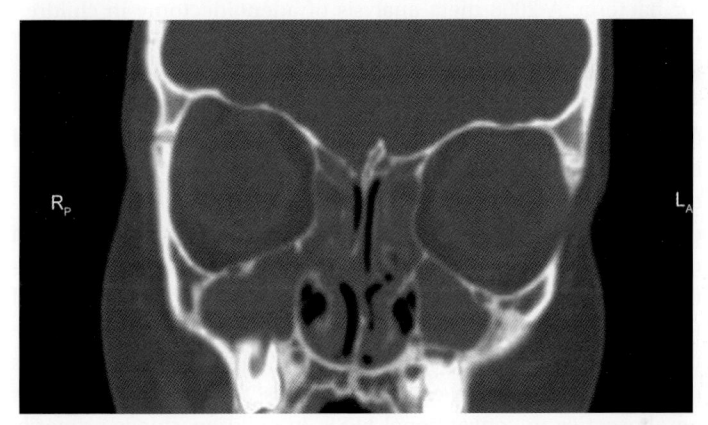

**Fig. 2:** Coronal computed tomography image of pediatric chronic rhinosinusitis.

The medical management of CRS has traditionally included combinations of antihistamines, decongestants, nasal saline irrigation, topical nasal steroids and oral antibiotics. Topical nasal steroids suppress mucosal inflammation and are therefore widely used in the treatment of CRS in children. Examples include fluticasone propionate or mometasone furoate, which is indicated for use in children 2 years of age and older. Evidence is limited but supports the use of both intranasal and systemic corticosteroids in the treatment of sinusitis, either alone or in combination with antibiotic therapy.[10,11] The use of topical nasal steroids is generally preferred for children with CRS because of their low systemic bioavailability. Systemic side-effects are therefore rare, with minor epistaxis the most commonly reported complication.[12] Antibiotics should be directed toward both aerobes and anaerobic organisms, particularly in patients with chronic sinusitis.[13] Evidence suggests that longer courses of antibiotic treatment (3–12 weeks) may be necessary to achieve any significant benefit.[14] In the absence of culture data, amoxicillin/clavulanate remains a good choice for first-line treatment, although antibiotic choices should also reflect the differences in possible pathogens in CRS. Long-term macrolide treatment (12 weeks) may also be of benefit in patients with CRS with low immunoglobulin E (IgE) levels.[15]

When medical therapy fails, children with persistent CRS should undergo surgical intervention. Adenoidectomy is the first line of surgical treatment for CRS in children, and is usually performed even before radiologic imaging with CT. Large adenoids may physically disrupt the normal clearance of the nasal cavity and sinuses, although adenoid tissue of any size is thought to act as a reservoir for bacteria. A 2008 meta-analysis of adenoidectomy in children with rhinosinusitis found an overall rate of clinical improvement of approximately 70%.[16]

In older (teenage) children, adenoid tissue tends to regress and become less clinically relevant. For this age group, functional endoscopic sinus surgery (FESS) is considered more frequently as an initial surgical procedure.[17] In children, the most common procedure is limited FESS and involves widening of the natural ostium of the maxillary sinus along with a limited or anterior ethmoidectomy. FESS is best considered as an adjuvant treatment to medical therapy, with the goal of improving sinus function by enlarging the natural ostia of the sinus. More recently, balloon dilation of sinus ostia known as balloon catheter sinuplasty has been reported as an alternative to conventional FESS. In children, this is primarily used for treatment of the maxillary sinus and has been described both alone and in combination with other procedures, such as adenoidectomy and ethmoidectomy.[18-20] Although safe, the potential complications of FESS include bleeding, infection, recurrence of disease, cerebrospinal fluid leak and orbital injury, including hematoma and loss of vision.

## EPISTAXIS

Epistaxis in children is a common disorder that is usually due to local irritation in Kiesselbach's area. The most common disorders underlying epistaxis are local inflammatory diseases, infections and trauma, including nose picking. Other diagnoses, including sinus and nasopharyngeal abnormalities, must be considered systematically. Epistaxis also may be the initial sign of serious systemic illness. Most children can be treated effectively with simple pressure to the alae and septum in case of infrequent epistaxis. Refractory bleeds may require progressively more aggressive measures. In case of recurrent epistaxis, application of antiseptic cream to the anterior septum may be effective. Silver nitrate cautery is an effective additional measure for which local anesthesia is usually required. Simultaneous bilateral cautery is not recommended owing to the possible increased risk of perforation of the septum.

Recurrences usually are prevented with medical management control of the local or systemic problem, but excessively frequent recurrences may require surgical correction.

## REFERENCES

1. Anand VK. Epidemiology and economic impact of rhinosinusitis. Ann Otol Rhinol Laryngol Suppl. 2004;193:3-5.
2. Lusk R. Pediatric chronic rhinosinusitis. Curr Opin Otolaryngol Head Neck Surg. 2006;14(6):393-6.
3. Benninger MS, Ferguson BJ, Hadley JA, et al. Adult chronic rhinosinusitis: definitions, diagnosis, epidemiology, and pathophysiology. Otolaryngol Head Neck Surg. 2003;129(3 Suppl):S1-32.
4. Ramadan HH. Pediatric sinusitis: update. J Otolaryngol. 2005;34 Suppl 1:S14-7.
5. Comstock RH, Lam K, Mikula S. Topical antibiotic therapy of chronic rhinosinusitis. Curr Infect Dis Rep. 2010;12(2):88-95.
6. Phipps CD, Wood WE, Gibson WS, et al. Gastroesophageal reflux contributing to chronic sinus disease in children: a prospective analysis. Arch Otolaryngol Head Neck Surg. 2000;126(7):831-6.
7. Bothwell MR, Parsons DS, Talbot A, et al. Outcome of reflux therapy on pediatric chronic sinusitis. Otolaryngol Head Neck Surg. 1999;121(3):255-62.
8. Carron J, Derkay C. Pediatric rhinosinusitis: is it a surgical disease? Curr Opin Otolaryngol Head Neck Surg. 2001;9:61-6.
9. American Academy of Pediatrics Subcommittee on Management of Sinusitis and Committee on Quality Improvement. Clinical practice guideline: management of sinusitis. Pediatrics. 2001;108(3):798-808.
10. Zalmanovici A, Yaphe J. Intranasal steroids for acute sinusitis. Cochrane Database Syst Rev. 2009;(4):CD005149.
11. Venekamp RP, Thompson MJ, Hayward G, et al. Systemic corticosteroids for acute sinusitis. Cochrane Database Syst Rev. 2011; (12):CD008115.
12. Skoner D. Update of growth effects of inhaled and intranasal corticosteroids. Curr Opin Allergy Clin Immunol. 2002;2(1):7-10.
13. Brook I. Chronic sinusitis in children and adults: role of bacteria and antimicrobial management. Curr Allergy Asthma Rep. 2005;5(6): 482-90.

14. Fokkens WJ, Lund VJ, Mullol J, et al. EPOS 2012: European position paper on rhinosinusitis and nasal polyps 2012. A summary for otorhinolaryngologists. Rhinology. 2012;50(1):1-12.
15. Adelson RT, Adappa ND. What is the proper role of oral antibiotics in the treatment of patients with chronic sinusitis? Curr Opin Otolaryngol Head Neck Surg. 2013;21(1):61-8.
16. Brietzke SE, Brigger MT. Adenoidectomy outcomes in pediatric rhinosinusitis: a meta-analysis. Int J Pediatr Otorhinolaryngol. 2008; 72(10):1541-5.
17. Ramadan HH. Surgical management of chronic sinusitis in children. Laryngoscope. 2004;114(12):2103-9.
18. Ramadan HH, McLaughlin K, Jospehson G, et al. Balloon catheter sinuplasty in young children. Am J Rhinol Allergy. 2010;24(1):e54-6.
19. Ramadan HH, Terrell AM. Balloon catheter sinuplasty and adenoidectomy in children with chronic rhinosinusitis. Ann Otol Rhinol Laryngol. 2010;119(9):578-82.
20. Sedaghat AR, Cunningham MJ. Does balloon catheter sinuplasty have a role in the surgical management of pediatric sinus disease? Laryngoscope. 2011;121(10):2053-4.

# *Index*

Page numbers followed by *f* refer to figure and *t* refer to table.

## A

Adenocarcinoma 75, 103
Adenoid cystic carcinomas 75
Adenoid hypertrophy 85*f*, 86
Agger nasi 12
 cell 21
Allergic rhinitis 41, 58, 87
Allergy 126
American Academy of Otolaryngology—Head and Neck Surgery 44
Amoxicillin 33
Angiofibromas 72
Angiotensin converting enzyme 80
 inhibitors 60
Anosmia 27, 43
Antibiotics 31, 48, 49
Antihistamines 32, 48
Atrophic rhinitis 82

## B

Bacterial acute rhinosinusitis 32*t*
Bacterial rhinosinusitis, acute 25
Bernoulli's principle 68

## C

Cavernous sinus thrombosis 52
Cefdinir 33
Cefixime 33
Cefuroxime 33
Cephalosporins 33
Cerebrovascular accident 118
Chandler's classification 51
Chandler's criteria 51
Charcot-Leyden crystals 47
Choanal atresia 70*f*, 87
Chronic rhinosinusitis, subtypes of 46*t*
Ciliary dyskinesia 126
Clarithromycin 33
Computed tomography 30, 63, 97
Concha bullosa 15, 17*f*, 70
Conductive disorders 3
Congenital midline nasal masses 71
Cough 43
Cranial nerve 5, 74
C-reactive protein 80
Cyclic adenosine monophosphate 3
Cystic fibrosis 126
Cytoplasmic antineutrophil cytoplasmic antibodies 80

## D

Dacrocystoceles 71
Dental pain 43
Doxycycline 33
Drug induced rhinitis 60

## E

Empty nose syndrome 83
Endoscopic arterial ligation 118
Endoscopic sinus surgery 48
Endoscopic sphenopalatine arterial ligation 118
Endovascular embolization 118
Enlarged inferior turbinates 86
Eosinophilia syndrome 61
Epistaxis 109, 128
Epstein-Barr virus 74
Esthesioneuroblastoma 76, 76*f*, 103
Ethmoid bulla 13, 10, 13
Ethmoid sinus 10, 17
Ethmoidal cells 112*f*

## F

Facial congestion 43
Facial pain 27, 43
Fatigue 27, 43
Fever 27, 32, 43
Fibro-osseous lesions and osteomas 72

Fluoroquinolones 33
Frontal intersinus septal cell 21
Frontal sinus 20, 21
Functional endoscopic
    sinus surgery 64, 128
Fungal infections 65

# G

Gastroesophageal reflux
    disease 126
Gram-positive
    Staphylococcus aureus 115
Granulomatosis 79

# H

Haemophilus
    influenzae 26, 46, 62, 125
Halitosis 43
Haller cell 15, 16*f*
Headache 27, 43
Hemophilia disorders 109
Hiatus semilunaris 14
Hormonal rhinitis 60
Human immunodeficiency
    virus (HIV) 60, 62
Human leukocyte antigen 74
Hypertrophied friable mucosa 79
Hyposmia 27, 43
Hypothyroidism 84

# I

Iatrogenic cerebrospinal fluid 17
Inferior turbinate
    hypertrophy 66, 68*f*
Infraorbital cell 26
Internal and external carotid
    arteries, branches of 110*f*
Internal carotid artery 112*f*
Internal maxillary artery,
    branches of 110, 110*f*
Invasive fungal sinusitis 88*f*
Inverted papilloma 71, 99
Juvenile angiofibroma 100
Juvenile nasopharyngeal
    angiofibroma 72, 73

# K

Kallmann syndrome 4
Keros classification 18*f*
Kiesselbach's area 128
Kiesselbach's plexus 110, 110*f*
Klebsiella ozaenae 82
Klebsiella pneumoniae 77

# L

Levofloxacin 33
Low temperature portable
    thermal cautery 116*f*

# M

Macrolides 33
Magnetic resonance
    angiography 72
Magnetic resonance
    imaging 30, 71, 97
Malaise 27
Malignant nasal neoplasms 101
Malignant tumor 76*f*
Maxillary and frontal sinus,
    postnatal development of 10*f*
Maxillary dental pain 27
Maxillary sinus 20, 21
Minor salivary gland tumors 75
Mohs excision 69
Moraxella catarrhalis 26, 63, 125
Moxifloxacin 33
Mucopurulent nasal discharge 27
Mucosal inflammation 57
Mucosal melanoma 76

# N

Nasal allergies 41
Nasal congestion/obstruction 27
Nasal cycle 7
Nasal decongestants 48
Nasal endoscopy 28
Nasal fontanelles 20
Nasal foreign body 87
Nasal fracture 86
Nasal masses 70
Nasal neoplasms 97, 98